Larry VandeCreek
Editor

Scientific and Pastoral Perspectives on Intercessory Prayer: An Exchange Between Larry Dossey, M.D. and Health Care Chaplains

Scientific and Pastoral Perspectives on Intercessory Prayer: An Exchange Between Larry Dossey, M.D. and Health Care Chaplains has been co-published simultaneously as *Journal of Health Care Chaplaincy*, Volume 7, Numbers 1/2 1998.

*Pre-publication
REVIEWS,
COMMENTARIES,
EVALUATIONS . . .*

"Scientific and Pastoral Perspectives on Intercessory Prayer: An Exchange Between Larry Dossey, M.D. and Health Care Chaplains* is a provocative book that addresses a difficulty encountered by many modern pastoral caregivers. The issue is intercessory prayer or, as Larry Dossey states, the 'effectiveness' of intercessory prayer. *Scientific and Pastoral Perspectives*, edited by Larry VandeCreek, takes the issue on. In the first part of the book Larry Dossey, a physician, presents evidence for the power of intercessory prayer. Dossey relies upon understandings of quantum physics and interpretations of consciousness that he and others make in quantum physics. Dossey's presentation for the effectiveness of intercessory prayer calls for a response. The second part of the book includes eight pastoral caregivers' responses to Dossey's research on prayer. The reactions run from those who favor what he has to say to those who are not moved by his words.

Dossey challenges ministers to take intercessory prayer seriously in their pastoral care ministry. His challenge reminds me of Paul Pruyser's challenge to ministers to assess people theologically and not just psychologically. In both cases the challenge comes from outside the ranks of the ordained clergy, but definitely from individuals sensitive and committed to religion. The basis for Dossey's argument for the effectiveness of intercessory prayer comes from science–not theology. 'It works,' he says and urges readers to take it seriously."

Howard W. Stone, PhD
Professor
Pastoral Theology
and Pastoral Counseling
Brite Divinity School
Texas Christian University

"**T**his book tackles that which appears to be a cultural and scientific paradigm shift. So, prayerful spirituality, scientifically validated, is seen by more people including their doctors as part of the healing process.

The book begins with a long chapter written by Larry Dossey, MD, who has emerged as a leader in alerting the medical and religious communities that there are 'healing words.' This chapter focuses his earlier *Healing Words* book in such a way that eight chaplains can respond to it constructively. Striking discussions arise in these responses about whether prayer is about faith in God or about participation in an efficacious process which sometimes can turn out well. Questions are asked: What is healing? How is it related to whatever the Absolute may be? How is quantum imaging useful in seeing the influencing energies in us and between us?

I found that many respondents had unforgettable stories to tell about their intercessions which seemed connected to astonishing improvements in health. Most seemed to be led into deeper mysteries by pondering these successes. They still don't understand how some of their intercessions did work.

Anyone who wonders about our

prayers and our needs will be drawn into these good dialogues involving scientific care and pastoral care."

Leland E. Elhard, PhD
Professor of Pastoral Theology
Trinity Lutheran Seminary
Columbus, Ohio

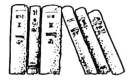

"**H**ealth care chaplains work in the front lines, daily experiencing firsthand the act of praying for patients in physical, emotional, mental, and spiritual pain. Often life-threatening pain. From this location in the trenches, chaplains also deal with the fear, rage, grief and remorse of the family and friends of the patient, even of the doctors and nurses. Falling on her or his head, and into their hearts, these chaplains carry the ministerial task, as Samuel put it, to bring the things of the people to God and the things of God to the people.

They welcome the article by Dossey that marshalls scientific research into the discernible effects of intercessory prayer. What is new to Dossey was known all along to the chaplains, as their different examples of patients eloquently attest. And they show, as well, their bewilderment and trust, their training and theological acumen that supports what Dossey discovers: that prayer makes a big difference in the health of the patient. Not only does it lower blood pressure, relieve stress, sometimes heal, and always help in pain management, as Dossey's helpful collection of research evidence indicates, intercessory prayer goes further, these chaplains say. It goes to an Other, an object of prayer, and hence distinguishes itself from any temptation to reduce intercession to a new 'spiritual prescription.' Intercessory prayer goes further than bringing us into awareness of our 'nonlocal consciousness,' as Dossey calls it, that acts freely in space and time and creates change in the physical world. Prayer for others opens a space in which we become conscious of an unconditional loving presence. Intercessory prayer creates a sacred space to which we all belong, so that we enter a community held in God, framed by God, as well as finding God present to each of us directly in unmediated presence.

Chaplains ask different questions than scientists. Less focused on results, they ask what the illness means for the one who is ill, and what are the symptoms that do not fit the diagnostic label, that might lead doctors and chaplains alike to another source of relief for the patient. Chaplains ask less about control and magical cure and more about how to enter the painful place the patient is, to set aside their own defenses in order to be with that person who is hurt and scared to such a degree that all of life seems to contract into a 'list of suffering.'

These chaplains welcome Dossey's urgent wish for conversations with them about the efficacy of prayer, while gently reminding him, and all of us, that the point of prayer is to enter into that loving presence that is there all the time urging our admittance through moving us to pray. Prayer also reveals theology. This group of interceding chaplains speak of a God who is there, whether we pray or not, who is present in unconditional forms of loving, who is boundless and beyond all our definitions and symbols. This God they focus on is one in relationship with us, connected to us and connecting us to each other, like a current, constantly, steadfastly moving us into its waters, so that it may flow through us all the more swiftly and deeply.

This book is helpful for those of us interested in conversations between science and religion, for those of us in pain, for those of us visiting ones we love in hospitals and nursing homes. The chaplains writing here represent different faiths, yet convey an openness to every faith because they all spring from the same mysterious author."

Ann Bedford Ulanov, MDiv, PhD, LHD
Christiane Brooks Johnson
Professor of Psychiatry and Religion
Union Theological Seminary, NYC;
Psychoanalyst in private practice

Scientific and Pastoral Perspectives on Intercessory Prayer: An Exchange Between Larry Dossey, M.D. and Health Care Chaplains

Scientific and Pastoral Perspectives on Intercessory Prayer: An Exchange Between Larry Dossey, M.D. and Health Care Chaplains has been co-published simultaneously as *Journal of Health Care Chaplaincy,* Volume 7, Numbers 1/2 1998.

Scientific and Pastoral Perspectives on Intercessory Prayer: An Exchange Between Larry Dossey, M.D. and Health Care Chaplains

Larry VandeCreek, DMin
Editor

Scientific and Pastoral Perspectives on Intercessory Prayer: An Exchange Between Larry Dossey, M.D. and Health Care Chaplains, edited by Larry VandeCreek, was simultaneously issued by The Haworth Pastoral Press, an imprint of The Haworth Press, Inc., under the same title, as a special issue of the *Journal of Health Care Chaplaincy,* Volume 7, Numbers 1/2 1998, Larry VandeCreek, Editor.

The Harrington Park Press
An Imprint of
The Haworth Press, Inc.
New York • London

ISBN 1-56023-113-0

Published by

The Harrington Park Press, 10 Alice Street, Binghamton, NY 13904-1580 USA

The Harrington Park Press is an imprint of The Haworth Press, Inc., 10 Alice Street, Binghamton, NY 13904-1580 USA.

Scientific and Pastoral Perspectives on Intercessory Prayer: An Exchange Between Larry Dossey, M.D. and Health Care Chaplains has been co-published simultaneously as *Journal of Health Care Chaplaincy,* Volume 7, Numbers 1/2 1998.

Cover design by Marylouise E. Doyle

Library of Congress Cataloging-in-Publication Data

Scientific and pastoral perspectives on intercessory prayer : an exchange between Larry Dossey, M.D. and health care chaplains / Larry VandeCreek, editor.
     p. cm.
     "Co-published simultaneously as Journal of health care chaplaincy, volume 7, numbers 1/2 1998."
     Includes bibliographical references and index.
     ISBN 0-7890-0518-2 (alk. paper).–ISBN 1-56023-113-0 (alk. paper)
     1. Intercessory prayer–Christianity. 2. Intercessory prayer–Comparative studies. 3. Medicine–Religious aspects. I. Dossey, Larry, 1940- . II. VandeCreek, Larry.
BV220.S32 1998
248.3'2–dc21   98-12323
                                                                                CIP

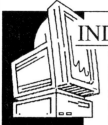

INDEXING & ABSTRACTING

Contributions to this publication are selectively indexed or abstracted in print, electronic, online, or CD-ROM version(s) of the reference tools and information services listed below. This list is current as of the copyright date of this publication. See the end of this section for additional notes.

- *Abstracts in Social Gerontology: Current Literature on Aging,* National Council on the Aging, Library, 409 Third Street SW, 2nd Floor, Washington, DC 20024

- *Abstracts of Research in Pastoral Care & Counseling,* Loyola College, 7135 Minstrel Way, Suite 101, Columbia, MD 21045

- *AgeLine Database,* American Association of Retired Persons, 601 E Street, NW, Washington, DC 20049

- *CNPIEC Reference Guide: Chinese National Directory of Foreign Periodicals,* P.O. Box 88, Beijing, People's Republic of China

- *Family Studies Database (online and CD/ROM),* National Information Services Corporation, 306 East Baltimore Pike, 2nd Floor, Media, PA 19063

- *HealthSTAR,* National Library of Medicine, 8600 Rockville Pike, Bethesda, MD 20894

- *Hospital and Health Administration Index,* American Hospital Association, One North Franklin, Chicago, IL 60606

- *Human Resources Abstracts (HRA),* Sage Publications, Inc., 2455 Teller Road, Newbury Park, CA 91320

- *INTERNET ACCESS (& additional networks) Bulletin Board for Libraries ("BUBL") coverage of information resources on INTERNET, JANET, and other networks.*
    - <URL:http://bubl.ac.uk/>
    - The new locations will be found under <URL:http://bubl.ac.uk/link/>.
    - Any existing BUBL users who have problems finding information on the new service should contact the BUBL help line by sending e-mail to <bubl@bubl.ac.uk>.
  The Andersonian Library, Curran Building, 101 St. James Road, Glasgow G4 0NS, Scotland

(continued)

- ***Leeds Medical Information,*** University of Leeds, Leeds LS2 9JT, United Kingdom

- ***Orere Source, The (Pastoral Abstracts),*** P.O. Box 362, Harbert, MI 49115

- ***Theology Digest (also made available on CD-ROM),*** St. Louis University, 3650 Lindell Boulevard, St. Louis, MO 63108

SPECIAL BIBLIOGRAPHIC NOTES

related to special journal issues (separates)
and indexing/abstracting

❑ indexing/abstracting services in this list will also cover material in any "separate" that is co-published simultaneously with Haworth's special thematic journal issue or DocuSerial. Indexing/abstracting usually covers material at the article/chapter level.

❑ monographic co-editions are intended for either non-subscribers or libraries which intend to purchase a second copy for their circulating collections.

❑ monographic co-editions are reported to all jobbers/wholesalers/approval plans. The source journal is listed as the "series" to assist the prevention of duplicate purchasing in the same manner utilized for books-in-series.

❑ to facilitate user/access services all indexing/abstracting services are encouraged to utilize the co-indexing entry note indicated at the bottom of the first page of each article/chapter/contribution.

❑ this is intended to assist a library user of any reference tool (whether print, electronic, online, or CD-ROM) to locate the monographic version if the library has purchased this version but not a subscription to the source journal.

❑ individual articles/chapters in any Haworth publication are also available through the Haworth Document Delivery Service (HDDS).

CONTENTS

ABOUT THE EDITOR

Larry VandeCreek, DMin, is Assistant Director of the Department of Pastoral Care and Clinical Associate Professor in the Departments of Family Medicine and Neurology at The Ohio State University Medical Center in Columbus, Ohio. Dr. VandeCreek is a member of numerous professional associations including the American Association of Marriage and Family Counselors, the College of Chaplains, Inc., the American Association of Pastoral Counselors, and the Association for Clinical and Pastoral Education. He has published many journal articles, abstracts, and is the author of *A Research Primer for Pastoral Care and Counseling* (Journal of Pastoral Care Publications, 1988). In addition, he is the Co-Editor of *The Chaplain-Physician Relationship* (1991) and Co-Author of *Ministry of Hospital Chaplains: Patient Satisfaction* (1997). Dr. VandeCreek received his Doctor of Ministry degree from Trinity Lutheran Seminary in Columbus, Ohio; his Master of Theology in Pastoral Counseling from the Columbia Theological Seminary in Atlanta, Georgia; and his Master of Divinity from Calvin Theological Seminary in Grand Rapids, Michigan.

Acknowledgments

As always, these materials did not mysteriously spring into existence. They required much thought, reflection, and the hard work of writing coherently. Thanks is due, therefore, to all the contributors. Special thanks is due to Larry Dossey, M.D. who provided the lead, original paper to which eight chaplains responded. He keeps a demanding schedule and we appreciate his extensive summary and review of his work.

Introduction

Larry VandeCreek, DMin

I write these lines to draw chaplains–and every reader–into thinking about intercessory prayer–what it is and what it is not. What can chaplains and patients expect from such intercessions? What does one think when the expected–or unexpected–happens during or after such prayers? Are there really unanswered–or answered–prayers? The attitudes and pastoral practice of every chaplain–every reader–implies answers to such questions.

Intercessory prayer and beliefs about it are central to ministry in Western culture. These prayers constitute the most frequent request of the dying, the sick, and the worried. They not only expect the chaplain to pray but to pray "effectively."

Furthermore, it seems that believers in every major religion engage in an activity that could be characterized as prayer, perhaps even intercessory prayer. I recently returned from India, having visited some Tibetan Hindu areas of the country with their prayer flags blown by the wind and prayer wheels turned by water. According to their theology, these prayers are offered as the wind blows and as the water turns the wheels. While these seem like strange practices for Western Christians and Jews, are we ready to claim that such practices do not constitute prayer, even intercessory prayer? Surely, our practices must seem strange to them.

In the lead article, Larry Dossey, M.D., summarizes his work on

[Haworth co-indexing entry note]: "Introduction." VandeCreek, Larry. Co-published simultaneously in *Scientific and Pastoral Perspectives on Intercessory Prayer: An Exchange Between Larry Dossey, M.D. and Health Care Chaplains* (ed: Larry VandeCreek) The Haworth Pastoral Press, an imprint of The Haworth Press, Inc., 1998, pp. 1-5; and: *Scientific and Pastoral Perspectives on Intercessory Prayer: An Exchange Between Larry Dossey, M.D. and Health Care Chaplains* (ed: Larry VandeCreek) Harrington Park Press, an imprint of The Haworth Press, Inc., 1998, pp. 1-5. Single or multiple copies of this article are available for a fee from The Haworth Document Delivery Service [1-800-342-9678, 9:00 a.m. - 5:00 p.m. (EST). E-mail address: getinfo@haworth.com].

1

prayer and challenges chaplains to think seriously about its place in their ministry. Eight chaplains respond. Some espouse complete endorsement of his ideas; most raise selected concerns, and others almost completely disagree with him.

Dossey's challenge represents far more than a concern about prayer. His work is based on a new way of thinking about the world and he asks about its implications for religious practice. This new approach which draws on quantum physics differs from the common-sense Ptolemaic world in which the sun rises and sets, the earth is firm under our feet, God is up in heaven or perhaps "in our hearts." It differs too from the Newtonian world in which God works through immutable natural laws. *The larger question that lies behind the concerns about intercessory prayer is, "Does this new physics make a difference in how we practice our faith, how we worship, and what we think about and expect from prayer?" Are we on the edge of revolutionary change in faith and practice or will this new physics not make any difference in our religious worlds?*

If quantum physics makes a difference, it will be another example of the interplay between physics and religion. In a helpful article titled "Spiritualities in a Post-Einsteinian Universe,"[1] David Toolan describes how religious changes followed modifications in the science of physics. He depicts Ignatius of Loyola as writing his Spiritual Exercises day after day at his desk in sixteenth century Rome and gazing at the stars from the roof of his residence at night. What was the meaning of this night-time gazing? Legend has it that these moments were his private spiritual exercises because, from his geocentric perspective, he thought of the stars as spiritually related to a world that was at the center of the universe. The heavens were one with his Ptolemaic world, the very stars themselves mediators of God's love and grace for the world and for him.

Then came Newton and the generations that followed saw these same stars as hard cold objects following a purely mechanical order. The stars were not tied to the earth, bringing a message of God's vast glory to humanity but rather bodies in vast space following cold and sterile laws of nature.

And now we have the physics of Einstein and his successors. We read about the mysterious behaviors of protons and electrons also in vast reaches of space–although now infinitesimally small. And this world of smallness is not so predictable, seemingly not so governed by immutable Newtonian laws. *Protons behave sometimes as particles and sometimes as waves. How do they know when to act like particles and when to act like waves? And it seems–according to Dossey and others–that equally unpredictable events sometimes occur at the more complex levels. A wide variety of enzymes as well as various fungi, yeasts, bacteria, cells in vitro, and plant seeds appear to respond positively to attention (or is it prayer?).* [2] *This is the world from which Dossey speaks, a world of non-local mind, of potent intentionality.*

History suggests that people involved in such shifting perspectives tend not to recognize the process of fundamental change; they are too close to the situation. They are also invested in the past. An old saying among scientists asks, "How does science change?" The answer: "It changes one funeral at a time." Likely, religious faith and practice change in the same way; the older generation dies and the younger one grows old having adopted the new perspective. Is that what is going on here, a fundamental shift in perspective, resisted by some and endorsed by others? Of course, it is also true that many clamor about world-shaking changes which then turn out to be more hype than reality. Perhaps our children or grandchildren will be able to answer more decisively and clearly.

In the meantime, the new physics as represented by Dossey raises interesting concerns about intercessory prayer which are important in their own right. I want to raise seven of these concerns here; keep these in mind as you read Dossey and the respondents.

First, is intercessory prayer sui generis? That is, is it truly different from everything else, not part of a larger phenomena? Is prayer in a classification category by itself or is it part of a larger category along with, for example, certain kinds of meditation and yoga?

Second, *intercessory* prayer is the focus here. What is its relationship to other forms of prayer, such as meditative prayer or those involving praise or thanksgiving? Are these forms of prayer part of some *sui generis* classification also?

Third, as you read Dossey and the chaplain respondents, ask yourself what constitutes convincing evidence in this discussion? That is, what kind of evidence moves you toward a decision about intercession? Is it the stories which describe personal experiences with intercession? Does careful, critical intellectual examination of prayer espoused by some respondents convince you? Does appealing to the Judeo-Christian Scriptures qualify as convincing evidence for you? The evidence cited in these pages is basic and applied, phenomenological and empirical, skeptical and believing. Dossey and the respondents vary widely in their choice of evidence. Some rely on a singular style of evidence; others are multi-faceted.

Fourth, as you read these materials, ask yourself, "What is God like for the writer?" Each writer, including Dossey, implies a God with certain characteristics. For some, God is very immanent and personal, active and intervening in ways continually creative; for others God is more distant, predictable, and rooted in natural laws. And various combinations of these characteristics are evident. These theological issues tend to be just beneath the surface of the text–and sometimes overtly present. The concern about miracles and unanswered (or efficacious) prayer tends to focus these concerns. Each respondent displays a theology.

Fifth, are the results of prayers linked in some way to the expectations or intentions of those who engage in them? Are these expectations or intentions the equivalent of faith? This becomes a particularly relevant concern when intercessions for healing take place. The linkage between the faith of the healer and the results is a common theme in the spiritual healing literature[3] and, of course, possesses Scriptural precedent (Matthew 21:22; Mark 11:24; James 5:13-20). If the faith of the pray-er is involved, then responses to intercession and possibility of healing differs with the individual chaplain. What are the implications of this for ministry, for pastoral care, for professional certification?

Sixth, what is the difference between an intercession and a wish? Or, are they the same? And if prayers for healing–or any other intercession–are only wishes, then they can easily become a sham. For example, what is the difference between an intercession for physical healing and for the local sports team to win the game? This concern is given increased weight because *proseuchomai*, one of the Greek scriptural words for "prayer," can also be translated as "wish."

Finally, I suggest you read these materials with both eyes open. That is, keep one eye on your own interior as you wrestle with Dossey and the respondents' comments. As always, your own subjective response will be important because it is the avenue into your pastoral practice. Be as clear as possible about what constitutes convincing evidence for you. The references used by each writer constitute a valuable resource you may wish to investigate further—and there is far more out there in the literature than is referenced here. W. Noel Brown has provided additional resources in the Current Contents Section near the end of this volume. At the same time, keep the other eye on the written responses because they reflect how chaplains as a profession regard the ministry of prayer. The respondents constitute a sample of what chaplains think and practice. It is evident that prayer is not a singular phenomena for these respondents; they think of and engage in prayer from many diverse points of view. And yet there are commonalities.

In summary, this book is devoted to exploring questions and concerns about intercessory prayer. And, as noted at the beginning, behind this rather concrete concern about prayer lies the deeper issues of how to think about and relate to the universe and God. These are not easy concerns to settle—and can not be settled once-and-for-all. It seems that Toolan points in an appropriate direction, however.

> If the military file conception of nature proposed by classical Newtonian physics shattered the sort of communion with the cosmos that Ignatius of Loyola could take for granted, post-Einsteinian cosmology begins to restore that communion. . . . The cosmos begins to appear to be a lot more irregular, even chaotic, than we had supposed, and the realm of life and human being appear to belong here. The poetry is back in nature.[1]

Our professional duties force us to think as clearly as possible about these issues so that we can practice responsibly. Read on!

REFERENCES

1. David S. Toolan. "Praying in a Post-Einsteinian Universe" *Cross Currents* Winter 1996-1997, 437-470.

2. For review of such studies see: Daniel Benor. "Survey of Spiritual Healing Research" in Larry Dossey *Healing Words* Harper, 1993.

3. For a current and comprehensive review of spiritual healing literature including comments from respondents and a rejoinder, see: David Aldridge. "Is there evidence for spiritual healing?" *Advances* 1993; 9(4):4-85.

ORIGINAL CONTRIBUTION

Prayer, Medicine, and Science:
The New Dialogue

Larry Dossey, MD

In 1996 I was invited to a large hospital in New York City. The day began with an address to the house staff in which I discussed the emerging scientific evidence for the effectiveness of intercessory prayer. I reviewed several of the salient experiments that had captured the attention of the medical profession and I summarized some of the studies that were currently in progress. Later in the day I met with the staff of the hospice department in a follow-up meeting. Before our discussion could begin, I was approached by a clergy person who was obviously quite disturbed. He worked full-time in the hospice area and devoted his life to offering spiritual

Larry Dossey is Executive Editor, *Alternative Therapies in Health and Medicine*, Santa Fe, NM 87501.

[Haworth co-indexing entry note]: "Prayer, Medicine, and Science: The New Dialogue." Dossey, Larry. Co-published simultaneously in *Journal of Health Care Chaplaincy* (The Haworth Pastoral Press, an imprint of The Haworth Press, Inc.) Vol. 7, No. 1/2, 1998, pp. 7-37; and: *Scientific and Pastoral Perspectives on Intercessory Prayer: An Exchange Between Larry Dossey, M.D. and Health Care Chaplains* (ed: Larry VandeCreek) The Haworth Pastoral Press, an imprint of The Haworth Press, Inc., 1998, pp. 7-37; and: *Scientific and Pastoral Perspectives on Intercessory Prayer: An Exchange Between Larry Dossey, M.D. and Health Care Chaplains* (ed: Larry VandeCreek) Harrington Park Press, an imprint of The Haworth Press, Inc., 1998, pp. 7-37. Single or multiple copies of this article are available for a fee from The Haworth Document Delivery Service [1-800-342-9678, 9:00 a.m. - 5:00 p.m. (EST). E-mail address: getinfo@haworth.com].

7

guidance and prayer for dying patients and to providing psychological and spiritual support for the hospice staff. *He said, "Look, I need to get something straight. I heard your lecture this morning—and if I understand you correctly, you're claiming that intercessory prayer actually works!"*

For a moment I was speechless and did not know how to respond. Although this man's life was immersed in prayer, he obviously harbored deep doubts about whether his prayers had any effect whatsoever. When confronted with evidence that intercessory prayer might actually be effective, he was astonished and confused. We chatted privately for a few moments, and I affirmed my earlier comments. I admired his honesty; most of us aren't as courageous as he was in expressing our doubts about prayer.

This experience confirmed my belief that even "true believers" often doubt, at some level of the mind, the effectiveness of prayer; and that religious professionals–hospital chaplains, pastoral counselors, ministers, priests, rabbis–*can be shocked to discover that science has something positive to say about prayer. I know that chaplains pray with patients and their families. I do not know how seriously they take that ministry. Some, perhaps many, may regard it as an obligation or as a purely religious performance in response to expectations. In this paper I intend to challenge chaplains to take prayer seriously, to take it seriously because of what science is discovering.* I will not review all the evidence because I have done so elsewhere.[1] Rather, I will discuss the various concerns that surround the issue of how prayer "works," particularly those relevant to clergy who provide pastoral care.

The reasons for the current ambivalence about prayer are complex, but are related to the stormy relations that have existed between science and religion for the past two centuries, particularly since Darwin. When battles between these two camps have arisen, religion usually has not fared well. As a result, many religious believers, including clergy, are understandably leery of what "science says" about their faith.

Another reason many religious persons object to the entry of science onto their turf is the stereotypical attitude toward science which most of us have developed during the process of becoming educated and socialized in twentieth-century America. The message that has been driven home to almost all of us in our colleges and universities is, "There are two ways to live your life. You can choose to be intellectual, rational, analytical, logical, and scientific; or, on the other hand, you can choose to be intuitive, spiritual, and religious. These two vectors of the psyche are incompatible and cannot be brought together; you cannot have it both ways." Most of us choose one path or the other, and suffer the rest of our life as a result of this artificial, schizophrenic split. The recent developments in prayer research show, however, that these choices are not incompatible. Science and spirituality can come together; we can have it both ways.

For the past five years I have had the opportunity to discuss science-and-prayer research with hospital chaplains, pastoral counselors, physicians, nurses, and other medical professionals in hospitals and medical schools across the United States. *My meetings with hospital-based spiritual counselors have invariably been a gratifying experience. Hospital chaplains and pastoral counselors are at home in medical environments where science dominates, and as a result they seem more cordial to science than do many other religious workers. While they may be initially surprised to discover that scientists have studied prayer empirically, they do not generally recoil from the idea, and many say their faith and belief in the power of prayer are empowered after learning about these developments.*

WHAT IS PRAYER?

It is important to address the definition of prayer because of the broad variety of prayers and pray-ers who have been studied in scientific experiments.

I have discussed this definition with thousands of Americans. *I have concluded that the most common image of prayer in our culture is something like this: "Prayer is talking aloud or to yourself, to a white, male, cosmic parent figure who prefers to be addressed in English."* This is, of course, an extremely limited and culturally conditioned view of prayer. It disenfranchises large proportions of the world's population, and non-whites in our own society who do not share this perspective. For example, many people believe that prayer can go beyond words to involve silence. For some, prayer is more a matter of being than doing–such as Thomas Merton, who once remarked that he prayed by breathing. Moreover, most people who pray worldwide are not white and they do not speak English (nor did Jesus or any of the founders of the world's major religions). Also, many people who pray are not fond of the idea of a male god or a personal god of any kind. Consider Buddhism, one of the world's great faiths. Buddhism is not a theistic religion, yet prayer is central to the Buddhist tradition. Buddhists offer their prayers to the universe, not to a personal god. Buddhism, therefore, violates most of the cultural assumptions we make about the nature of prayer. Shall we inform Buddhists and others who differ from our cultural norm that they aren't really praying?

In the following discussion I want to employ a deliberately broad and ambiguous definition of prayer: "Prayer is communication with the Absolute." This definition is inclusive, not exclusive; it affirms religious tolerance; and it invites people to define for themselves what "communication" is, and who or what "the Absolute" may be. This definition is broad enough to include people of the various faiths who have participated as subjects in prayer research.

I now narrow the definition to intercessory prayer. "Intercessory" comes from the Latin *inter,* "between," and *cedere,* "to go." *Intercessory prayer is, therefore, a go-between—an effort to mediate on behalf of, or plead the case of, someone else. Intercessory prayer is often called "distant" prayer, because the individual being prayed for is often remote from the person who is praying.*

SURVEYING THE FIELD

How much experimental data supports intercessory prayer? There is a significant difference of opinion. If one performs an electronic database search using "prayer" as a key word, one will probably retrieve around a half-dozen studies of dubious quality. On the other hand, physician Daniel J. Benor has written a four-volume work, *Healing Research*[2] (the first two volumes of which have been published), which cites nearly 150 studies in this field, many of which are of excellent quality and over half of which show statistically significant results.

Part of the problem in identifying work in this field is the lack of agreement on language. Many researchers shy away from using the word "prayer" in favor of a more neutral term such as "distant intentionality." Even though their experiment may actually involve prayer, they often do not use this term in the titles of their papers. If their subjects pray, the researcher may say instead that the subject "concentrated" or applied "mental effort" to produce the effect being studied, or they may use terms such as "mental healing," "psi healing," or "spiritual healing" to describe their work.

Perhaps we should not be too critical of researchers on this point. Research in the distant effects of consciousness is generally considered to be the domain of parapsychology. This field is sufficiently controversial without adding the furor surrounding the concept of distant, intercessory prayer. But the aversion of experimenters to using "prayer" comes with a price–the difficulty of identifying prayer-and-healing studies, and the underestimation of the number of prayer experiments that exists.

ABOUT PRAYER AND PARAPSYCHOLOGY

Many religious persons are exceedingly uncomfortable about "parapsychology," and they deplore the practice of parapsychologists of equating prayer with mental intentionality, focused attention, concentration, or even meditation. They often feel that parapsychologists dishonor prayer and are disrespectful of the spiritual traditions in which prayer is embedded. I sympathize with these reservations; but after exploring prayer and parapsychology for several years, I feel that a clean separation between these fields does not exist and is impossible to achieve without resorting to the cultural limitations noted above. In parapsychology experiments, individuals often actually pray or enter a sacred, reverential, prayer-like state of mind to accomplish their task. On the other hand, when people pray, they often have paranormal experiences such as telepathy, clairvoyance, or precognition. Anyone doubting this would do well to read philosopher Donald Evans' scholarly work, *Spirituality and Human Nature*,[3] or historian Brian Inglis' classic book *Natural and Supernatural: A History of the Paranormal*.[4]

Fortunately, the longstanding antipathy between religion and parapsychology appears to be diminishing. The *Journal of Religion and Psychical Research*,[5] published in the United States and *The Christian Parapsychologist*,[6] published in Great Britain, are notable examples of bridge-building between these fields. The latter publication was begun in 1953 by a group of British clergy and laymen who were "convinced that psychical phenomena [have] great relevance to the Christian faith, both in life and death . . . [but that] psychical studies are as likely to lead to harm as to good if pursued outside the realms of the spiritual life . . . through the practice of prayer, worship and service to [our] fellow creatures."

As further evidence of the emerging religion-and-parapsychology dialogue, Michael Stoeber, Assistant Professor in the Department of Religion and Religious Education at The Catholic University of America, and Hugo Meynell, Professor in the Department of Religious Studies at the University of Calgary, have co-edited a critically acclaimed book, *Critical Reflections on the Paranormal*,[7] that examines issues of mutual interest to both parapsychology and religion.

PRAYER AND PSI IN THE LAB

As a single example of how parapsychology (often called "psi") and prayer are difficult if not impossible to keep separate, consider a study by Haraldsson and Thorsteinsson in which subjects attempted mentally to cause increases in the growth rate of yeast cultures. The title of the paper, "Psychokinetic Effects on Yeast: An Exploration Experiment,"[8] gives no hint that spiritual healers and prayer were involved. The researchers recruited seven subjects–two spiritual healers who used prayer, one physician who employed spiritual healing and prayer in his practice, and four students with no experience or particular interest in healing. The subjects were asked to "direct their healing effects" to increase the growth of yeast in 120 test tubes. The study was well designed and employed appropriate controls. The results indicated that "mental concentration or intention" indeed affected the growth of the yeast. The bulk of the scoring was done by the two spiritual healers and the physician, which yielded a p value of <0.00014, meaning that the odds against a chance result were less than 14 in 100,000. In contrast, the students, who had little interest in either prayer or healing, scored at chance levels.

The title of this paper suggests that it was a study in parapsychology and psychokinesis ("mind over matter"), but a closer look shows that it was clearly an experiment in the effects of prayer. Because of its title, however, a survey of the prayer-and-healing literature would probably not identify this study. This experiment is a typical example of why the boundaries between prayer and experimental parapsychology are artificial.

LOVE IN THE LAB

There are other reasons for associating prayer and parapsychology. Subjects in parapsychology experiments often experience feelings that are central to prayer such as love, empathy, compassion, and a sense of connectedness, oneness, and unity with the object they are attempting to influence.[9] Robert G. Jahn, former dean of engineering at Princeton University and the director of the Princeton Engineering Anomalies Research Laboratory, has recently begun to address the role of love in the mental interaction of subjects with electronic, random event generators and other physical devices. One of their most successful subjects said, "I simply fell in love with the machine."[10] Experiences such as these are extremely common in psi subjects. In them, love seems to function as a form of intercession—literally, a go-between—that unites the subject and the object being influenced. If love is crucial to the success of psi experiments, and if "God is love," then the Almighty appears to be less nervous than some believers about entering the parapsychology lab.

Both religionists and parapsychology researchers should pay closer attention to the actual experiences of successful subjects in psi experiments. If they did so, they might see that actual prayer or a sense of prayerfulness manifesting as love, reverence, and felt unity permeates the many trials of distant intentionality that exist in the parapsychology literature. These experiences imply that a silent element of sacredness exists in the psi lab that is not often acknowledged. If this reverential quality of psi research was recognized, it would expand the science-and-prayer literature to an immense degree.

On balance, therefore, the classic parapsychology studies which mention prayer explicitly[11] are but the tip of a gigantic iceberg, and the data supporting the role of prayer is more vast than we have imagined.

PRAYER EXPERIMENTS AS SACRED SCIENCE

A common complaint against prayer experiments in general is that these studies "test God" and are therefore blasphemous. The blasphemy argument has even been used by skeptical scientists as a reason to oppose the empirical testing of prayer.[12] In contrast, many scientists believe that the experimental approach can be a form of worship. For example, the Jesuit priest, scholar, and paleontologist Pierre Teilhard de Chardin said that research is the highest form of adoration. All the researchers I know who are currently investigating the effects of intercessory prayer embody a sense of sacredness in their work, as if they are treading on holy ground.

STUDIES HUMAN AND NONHUMAN

Studies in distant, prayerful intentionality involving living systems involve both humans and nonhumans. William G. Braud, director of research at the Institute of Transpersonal Psychology in Palo Alto, reports, ". . . persons have been able to influence, mentally and at a distance, a variety of biological target systems including bacteria, yeast colonies, motile algae, plants, protozoa, larvae, woodlice, ants, chicks, mice, rats, gerbils, cats, and dogs, as well as cellular preparations (blood cells, neurons, cancer cells) and enzyme activity. In human 'target persons,' eye movements, gross motor movements, electrodermal activity, plethysmographic activity, respiration, and brain rhythms have been influenced."[13] As already mentioned, physician Daniel J. Benor has identified around 150 of these studies in his four-volume analysis of this area.[14]

Many people are puzzled how anyone could love bacteria, fungi, germinating seeds, rats, or mice sufficiently to pray for them. This attitude is quite widespread, even among devout practitioners of prayer. I recently received a letter from a woman in Italy. Her cat had been run over by an auto and was paralyzed in its hind limbs. When she asked the local friars if they would pray for her cat's healing, they told her it was fruitless to pray for animals because they did not have souls and could not respond to prayer. She was heartbroken to consider that her beloved cat was outside the reach of prayer. It is paradoxical that this opinion originated not far from Assisi, the home of St. Francis, who would probably have been appalled at the discriminatory attitude of the modern friars toward animals.

Susan J. Armstrong, Professor of Philosophy and Women's Studies at Humboldt State University, has extensively examined these questions in a provocative essay, "Souls in Process: A Theoretical Inquiry into Animal Psi." She notes that Pope John Paul II has recently reaffirmed the early Christian doctrine that animals have souls, which presumably implies that they are fit subjects for prayer. She notes, "In a homily at the Vatican in 1989 the Pope quoted Ps. 104, in which animals are said to have the breath of life from God, and called for 'solidarity with our smaller brethren.' "[15]

Still, the use of nonhumans in prayer studies remains a stumbling block for many people. Yet other cultures are not as troubled on this point. I have visited temples in India dedicated to the worship of rats, in which people pray for these creatures and lovingly offer them food. For their part, the rats seem appreciative. If this practice seems bizarre, we might bear in mind that we also worship mice in our culture without realizing it. The major icon of the Disney empire is a mouse. Each year, millions of American families undertake expensive pilgrimages to two major shrines—Disneyland and Disneyworld—to express their devotion. And every night, thousands of American children offer bedtime prayers that their parents will reward them with a visit to the Magic Kingdom, whose ruler is a small rodent.

Part of the resistance to praying for animals in formal experiments is due to the growing gulf between animals and humans that has developed with increasing urbanization. When America was more rural, prayer for animals was widespread and seemed natural. *I grew up on a farm in Texas; and although we never prayed for mice or bacteria, we prayed incessantly for cows, pigs, horses, germinating seeds and growing plants, as do farmers worldwide.* Even in urban America, millions of vegetarians feel so intimately connected with animals that they find it unthinkable to eat them. Many pray and work diligently for the welfare of animals and for the preservation of endangered species. Many veterinarians consider it quite natural to pray for their patients.[16] I have attended churches in the United States who help place homeless animals, and which feature "pet prayer" as part of the worship program. Therefore, the feelings of compassion, love, and bondedness toward nonhumans, although highly variable, are nonetheless widespread, and support the idea that the power of prayer can be studied experimentally in nonhumans and humans alike.

ARE EXPERIMENTS THAT INVOLVE MICROORGANISMS RELEVANT TO PRAYER?

As we have seen, some experiments deal with prayer not for cuddly pets such as cats and dogs, but with invisible microorganisms. Many people believe these studies cannot possibly involve prayer because there is no biblical injunction to pray for or against microbes. But, of course, the Bible is mute on this question because the concepts of bacteria, fungi, yeast, and viruses did not exist in biblical times. Therefore, we must interpret for ourselves whether or not it is fitting to apply prayer to these creatures.

There are indirect biblical sanctions to pray both for and against microbes. For example, when we pray for the sick, as we are instructed to do, this often includes those suffering from infections. A prayer for someone with an infectious disease is a prayer against the microorganisms involved, whether we realize it or not. Likewise, when we pray that our food, which is never sterile, be blessed, we are presumably asking that the bacteria it contains be put out of commission. *A sanction to pray for microbes can be found in the Lord's Prayer. When we pray for our daily bread, this presumably includes praying for the yeast cells that make it rise.*

Microbes are not insignificant when compared to humans, because without them human life could not exist. All ecological systems are microbe-dependent. How could prayer involving microorganisms be trivial, when our life is inextricably linked to theirs?

BUT IS IT PRAYER?

When confronted with experimental evidence that prayer can indeed enhance or retard microbial growth, some religionists dedicated to an anthropocentric view of prayer resort to a last-ditch objection—that these effects are not really due to prayer but to "mind over matter" or some "mental force" (although they have never been able to clarify what this force might be). Others condemn these effects as "the work of the devil" and let it go at that. Some engage in *ad hominem* attacks on the pray-ers, claiming that anyone who would be willing to engage in such an experiment must be trying to demonstrate their personal power instead of God's, which is further evidence that these studies are corrupt and blasphemous.

Perhaps the strongest evidence that these studies involve genuine, authentic prayer is the fact that respected spiritual healers often serve as the subjects, as we have already seen in the Haraldsson and Thorsteinsson experiment.[17] As a further example, consider a study involving the well-known spiritual healer Olga Worrall, who for years conducted prayer-based healing services at The New Life Clinic at Baltimore's Mt. Washington United Methodist Church.[18] Mrs. Worrall was revered by all who knew her as a humble servant of God. On one occasion she accepted the invitation of physicist Elizabeth A. Rauscher and microbiologist Beverly A. Rubik to participate in a laboratory experiment involving bacteria. The study originally called for Worrall to inhibit bacterial activity in a particular phase of the experiment. When she objected to using prayer to harm God's creatures, the study was redesigned to allow her to help, not hurt, the microorganisms by protecting them from the killing effects of antibiotics. The results showed that she was able to do so.[19] It is difficult to dismiss this study as not involving genuine prayer, with which Mrs. Worrall was intimately familiar.

Are the pray-ers in these experiments glorifying themselves instead of the Almighty, as often charged? Are they putting their ego first? For all I know, this objection may have merit in some cases. But if it does, it surely applies to prayers offered in church as well in the laboratory. We cannot fully know the heart of another person. This fact should make us hesitant to pass judgment on the sincerity of the prayers of others, whether they take place inside or outside the lab.

THE MOST FAMOUS PRAYER STUDY

The most celebrated twentieth-century prayer study involving humans was published in 1988 by physician Randolph Byrd,[20] a staff cardiologist at University of California at San Francisco School of Medicine. Byrd randomized 393 patients in the coronary care unit at San Francisco General Hospital to either a group receiving intercessory prayer or to a control group. Intercessory prayer was offered by groups outside the hospital; they were not instructed how often to pray, but only to pray as they saw fit. In this double-blind study, in which neither the patients, physicians, nor nurses knew who was receiving prayer, the prayed-for patients did better on several counts. There were fewer deaths in the prayer group (although this factor was not statistically significant); they were less likely to require endotracheal intubation and ventilator support; they required fewer potent drugs including diuretics and antibiotics; they experienced a lower incidence of pulmonary edema; and they required cardiopulmonary resuscitation (CPR) less often.

Byrd's study illustrates some of the difficulties in studying the effects of intercessory prayer in humans.[21] In any controlled study, the control group ideally should not receive the treatment being tested, whether the treatment is a drug, prayer, or something else. But in prayer studies involving humans who are seriously ill, subjects in the control group may pray for themselves, or their loved ones and friends may pray for them—"the problem of extraneous prayer." Even though the degree of outside prayer may equalize between the treatment and control groups, a major problem remains. If both groups are prayed for, the experiment becomes not a test of prayer versus no prayer, but a test of the degree or the amount of prayer. "It could be that the efforts of these strangers [who are recruited to prayer for the 'prayer treatment' group] will be swamped by the heart-felt prayers of those directly involved with the patients," says professor of physics Russell Stannard of the Open University in England.[22] If so, both groups might benefit equally from prayer, with no significant differences detectable between them. In technical jargon this is called reduction of the "effect size" between the two groups. This can be a vexing methodological problem, because it means that prayer can appear ineffective even when it worked. Although this problem can be dealt with through sophisticated research methods, it is a major obstacle in perhaps all the prayer studies involving sick humans.

Researchers have considered ways of overcoming the problem of self-prayer by subjects in the control group—for example, using sick infants or newborns, or unconscious, brain-damaged adults, who do not pray for themselves. But this still does not eliminate the confounding effect of prayer by loved ones and friends.

These research difficulties can be completely overcome if nonhumans instead of humans are used as subjects. If bacteria are employed, for example, the organisms in the control group presumably do not pray for themselves, nor do their fellow bacteria pray for them. These simple facts are but one reason why it is possible to achieve great precision in nonhuman prayer studies, and why the effect sizes of these studies often dwarf those seen in human experiments.

Although the design of Byrd's study could have been improved, he deserves immense credit for undertaking the experiment. He established a principle–that distant, intercessory prayer can be studied like a drug in humans, in a controlled fashion, in a sophisticated medical environment. Byrd's contribution is monumental–not because it was the first prayer study (many others preceded it), but because it captured the public's attention and helped break a taboo in this area of medical research.

PRAYER IN THE LAB: A BENEDICTINE PERSPECTIVE

Many people believe prayer is more appropriate to religious ceremony than to the nitty-gritty world of scientific experimentation, as if prayer is wrapped in some celestial halo and is easily sullied when used for secular purposes. The Benedictine Order would probably have disagreed with this restriction. They chose as their ancient motto, "Orare est laborare, laborare est orare"–"To pray is to work, to work is to pray." What if one works in a lab? Can't prayer be part of lab work, as the Benedictine attitude implies? Why should prayer be genuine in church or synagogue but bogus in the lab?

Sometimes a slight shift in perspective can help us see how prayer can be used in the most unlikely situations. Jean Kinkead Martine describes a conversation between two Zen monks. Both were prodigious smokers and they were concerned whether it was permissible to smoke during their prayer time. They decided individually to ask the abbott of the monastery his opinion and then compare notes. One said, "I asked 'Is it permitted to smoke while praying?' and I was severely reprimanded." The other said, "But I asked, 'Is it permitted to pray while smoking,' and the abbot gave me a pat of encouragement."[23]

Martine says, "To pray while typing, while answering the phone–would it require, a very different way of praying; a way that Zen monks must come to through their training–something like that wordless beseeching one discovers in trying to guide a car along an icy road or in performing any exacting piece of work under all but impossible conditions?"[24] I like Martine's image—"that wordless beseeching . . . in trying to guide a car along an icy road." Subjects in studies in distant intentionality use a kind of "wordless beseeching." They try to coax, nudge, help, and somehow guide the experiment toward a certain outcome, often through prayer.

In my book *Healing Words*[25] I advanced the concept of "prayerfulness" to describe how prayer can become a natural part of our daily tasks. Prayerfulness is more a matter of being than doing. I discovered that this makes sense to a lot of physicians. An eminent surgeon wrote me that after his medical and surgical training he abandoned prayer and never formally prayed for his patients. Yet, after thinking about the concept of prayerfulness, he realizes that he prays continually for his patients through his feelings of empathy, caring and compassion for them—that, in fact, surgery for him is a continual exercise in prayer.

OBJECTIONS TO PRAYER RESEARCH: THE RELIGIOUS COMMUNITY

When I began to research the experiments that have been done in prayer, I believed that religious people who believed in prayer would be uniformly delighted to discover the scientific evidence that prayer worked. I was, therefore, surprised to discover that some religious groups responded to these findings with vehement objections. There were two main reasons.

One, already mentioned, is the belief that prayer experiments are done by unbelieving heretics bent on "testing God." I believe this is a mischaracterization of researchers involved in prayer, and is irrational as well. Does anyone really believe that a die-hard skeptic would spend valuable time and scarce research funds investigating a phenomenon which he bitterly opposed in the first place? Researchers choose topics toward which they feel cordial, not those they consider fallacious.

In fact, the attitude of most prayer researchers appears to be precisely the opposite of "testing God." One prayer researcher says that when she performs a prayer experiment, she is not setting a trap but opening a window through which the Almighty can manifest. Another prayer experimenter imagines that arranging a prayer experiment is like preparing an elegant meal in his home. When the table is set and the food is served, he opens the door of his house and waits patiently to see if anyone shows up. If a guest appears (if the experiment works), the meal was a success; if not, it's back to the drawing board to design a more inviting situation. Again, I know most of the researchers in this area, and I believe they are some of the most spiritually grounded people I have ever met. I believe all of them would agree that one can conduct prayer experiments with a profound sense of sacredness, reverence, and respect.

The biblical injunction against "testing God" may not have referred to the randomized, double-blind, controlled lab experiment, since this procedure did not then exist. Might the Almighty actually want to be tested in this particular way? The British physicist Russell Stannard states, "I know that it says in the Bible that we should not put God to the test, but I can't think that God would take offence. He will probably be tickled that we are using our God-given sense of curiosity."[26]

I discovered that there was a more subtle objection against prayer experiments from some religious groups. They seemed troubled by the absence of any correlation between the effect of the prayer and the religious affiliation of the person praying. *The prayer experiments showed clearly that no religion has a monopoly on prayer, and that prayer is a universal phenomenon belonging to all of humankind and not to any specific religion.* Some fundamentalist groups found this implication offensive, and chose to condemn all the experimental evidence favoring prayer in an attempt to preserve their own sense of specialness.

OBJECTIONS TO PRAYER RESEARCH: THE SCIENTIFIC COMMUNITY

There appears to be a growing attitude within the scientific community that intercessory prayer can be researched just as any other phenomenon, as evidenced by the studies now in progress at several academic centers. Yet opposition from scientists exists, most of it coming from a small but vocal minority.

Those who oppose the idea of intercessory prayer do so mainly because of the prevalent belief that human consciousness can be generally equated with the workings of the brain, which means that the effects of the mind are confined to the physical brain and body.

According to this view, consciousness cannot in principle cause things to happen at a distance, whether of its own accord or by acting through a transcendent agency. From this standpoint, intercessory prayer raises the old bugaboo of "spooky action at a distance" and is considered outrageous.

Perhaps no issue within science evokes such extreme emotional responses as "mental action at a distance." For example, G. R. Price, an avowed foe of parapsychology, writing in the prestigious journal *Science,* said, "Not 1000 experiments with ten million trials and by 100 separate investigators giving total odds against chance of one-thousandth to 1 [could make me accept ESP]"[27]–or, presumably, distant, intercessory prayer. Hermann von Helmholtz (1821-94), a towering figure in physics in the nineteenth century, commented, *"I cannot believe it. Neither the testimony of all the Fellows of the Royal Society, nor even the evidence of my own senses would lead me to believe in the transmission of thought from one person to another independently of the recognized channels of sensation. It is clearly impossible."*[28] An additional example of this attitude came from a peer-reviewer of a prestigious scientific journal who was asked to evaluate a paper dealing with these matters. He commented, "This is the kind of thing that I would not believe in even if it existed."[29]

If distant mental phenomena and intercessory prayer are as nutty as some skeptics insist, why are an increasing number of prominent scientists investigating them? According to one theory, the researchers are either incompetent, are liars and cheats, or their brains aren't working right. This view was expressed by G. R. Price in the same article in *Science*: "My opinion concerning the findings of [these researchers] is that many of them are dependent on clerical and statistical errors and unintentional use of sensory clues, and that all extrachance results not so explicable are dependent on deliberate fraud or mildly abnormal mental condition."[30]

Probably all skeptics who are opposed to intercessory prayer are also opposed to the field of parapsychology, which deals with distant mental phenomena such as telepathy, clairvoyance, precognition, and psychokinesis. Indeed, skeptics oppose intercessory prayer and parapsychology for virtually the same reasons. They seem convinced that these phenomena so profoundly violate the laws of physics that they should be dismissed a priori. The eminent physicist Gerald Feinberg disagrees. Speaking of precognition–knowing something before it happens, which is probably the most challenging parapsychological event of all, and which bears a strong resemblance to prophecy–he says, "[I]f such phenomena indeed occur, no change in the fundamental equations of physics would be needed to describe them."[31] In addition, psychologist Paul Meehl and philosopher of science Michael Scriven have pointed out that many of the objections of skeptics toward distant mental intentionality rest on two highly questionable assumptions: that current scientific knowledge is complete and that ESP–and, we might add, intercessory prayer–necessarily conflicts with it.[32] Epidemiologist Jeffrey S. Levin, one of the foremost authorities on the correlations between religious practice and health, has advanced a theoretical model of how prayer heals that places this phenomenon fully within scientific respectability.[33]

The skeptical complaint that the distant effects of prayer simply can not happen because there is no accepted theory within science that would permit them is a peculiar objection. In science, the demonstration of empirical facts often precedes the development of an accepted, explanatory theory. An example from the history of medicine is the practice of washing one's hands before delivering babies or doing surgery. When Semmelweiss, in 1848, produced overwhelming evidence for the effectiveness of handwashing, his colleagues could not believe it. At that time the germ theory of disease did not exist and the idea of handwashing was considered preposterous. Semmelweiss was hounded out of Vienna, fled to Budapest, and finally committed suicide. A fully developed theory supporting handwashing came later and Semmelweiss was vindicated. Similar events took place in America. When the Boston physician Oliver Wendell Holmes also proposed handwashing and scrupulous cleanliness to his colleagues in Boston in 1843, he was violently opposed by the prominent Philadelphia obstetricians Hodge and Meigs.[34]

Events such as these show that it is possible for medical science to progress in a thick theoretical fog. Consider many therapies that are now commonplace, such as the use of aspirin, quinine, colchicine, and penicillin. For a long time we knew that they worked before we knew how. Today we are in a similar situation with intercessory prayer: data suggesting its effectiveness has arisen prior to the development of a generally accepted theory. This should alarm no one who has the meagerest knowledge of how medicine has progressed through the ages.

Sometimes scientific facts are accepted but never explained. In the 1600s, when Newton invoked the idea of universal gravity, he was attacked by his contemporaries as surrendering to mysticism. They disapproved of the mysterious force of gravity because Newton could not explain why bodies behaved in accordance with his proposed laws, or how physical bodies could act at a distance on one another. "This sort of worry no longer bothers us, but not because we have answered it," observes philosopher Eugene Mills of Virginia Commonwealth University.[35] We've simply gotten used to the idea. So it may turn out with intercessory prayer.

DEBUNKING THE DEBUNKERS

In addition to charges of sloppy methodology, deliberate deception, and having abnormal brains, skeptics often charge that these studies are done by rogue scientists functioning outside academic settings, that the studies are not published in peer-reviewed journals, that negative findings are not reported (the "file drawer effect"), and that no studies have been replicated. Most of these perennial complaints are blatantly false.

As we've seen, the evidence for intercessory prayer is not limited to a single type of organism; "targets" include a spectrum of creatures such as humans, a variety of animals, bacteria, fungi, healthy and cancerous tissue from both humans and animals, and enzyme preparations. The variety of targets is immensely important. Critics claim that these effects are due only to psychological processes such as suggestion and expectation–the placebo response. However, the fact that nonhumans are used in these studies refutes this argument–unless skeptics wish to maintain that microbes, enzymes, and cells have an emotional life similar to human beings.

Current researchers in the field of distant intentionality and prayer often hold faculty appointments at prestigious institutions, including major medical schools. Many of their studies embody the highest scientific standards including proper randomization and control procedures, and many have been replicated. Moreover, it is the most rigorous studies, which involve nonhumans, which gener-

ally produce the most robust and significant results–exactly opposite the charge of most skeptics.

This does not mean that all the studies in this field are perfect.
The quality of experiments varies in any field of science, and this
area is no exception. In assessing this or any other field, one should
look at the very best studies and try to discern the general direction
in which they point. This contrasts with the strategy of many skeptics, who often cite the very worst study they can find and general-
ize to condemn the entire field.

There is no single "killer study" that makes an irrefutable case
for intercessory prayer. In this field, as in most other areas of medical science, it is the concatenation or linking together of many
strands of evidence that builds the case, not what any single study
shows.

*The major criticisms against distant mental phenomena, includ-
ing intercessory prayer, have in my opinion been firmly refuted.*
This is not the place to address these issues in detail; I have done so
elsewhere[36,37] as have many respected scholars. For a review of
these refutations, I suggest the following sources:

- Dean I. Radin and Roger D. Nelson. "Evidence for consciousness-related anomalies in random physical systems." *Foundations of Physics* 1989; 19:1499-1514.
- Dean I. Radin. "A field guide to skepticism." *The Conscious
  Universe* (San Francisco: HarperEdge), 1997, in press.
- Jessica Utts. "An assessment of the evidence for psychic functioning." *Journal of Scientific Exploration.* 1996; 10(1):3-30.
- Charles Honorton. "Rhetoric over substance: the impoverished
  state of skepticism." *Journal of Parapsychology.* 1993: 57(2):
  191-214.
- Mark B. Woodhouse. "Why CSICOP is losing the war." *Paradigm Wars* (Berkeley, CA: Frog, 1996),116-21.

DOES PRAYER KILL?

As prayer experiments have become popularized by the media, a
particular charge of skeptics seems to be gaining in popularity–that
it is dangerous to speak about the evidence favoring intercessory

prayer. Doing so will induce hoards of sick individuals to take up prayer, use it exclusively, and abandon the use of "real medicine," with lethal consequences. This worry appears irrational. Surveys from the Gallup organization and the National Opinion Research Center of the University of Chicago reveal that the vast majority of Americans (80 to 90 percent) already pray regularly; they don't "take up prayer" when sick. Neither are they likely to bail out of orthodox medicine when they confront a health crisis. Although certain religions such as Christian Science do favor the exclusive use of prayer during illness, surveys consistently show that the vast majority of Americans are extremely pragmatic when they are sick. They generally employ both standard and complementary methods of health care, including prayer, and do not opt for a single approach.[38,39]

THE CHANGING FACE OF SKEPTICISM

Some of the best-informed skeptics about distant mental effects seem recently to be taking a defensive posture. *As skeptical psychologist Ray Hyman acknowledges, "The case for psychic functioning seems better than it ever has been. The contemporary findings . . . do seem to indicate that something beyond odd statistical hiccups is taking place. I . . . have to admit that I do not have a ready explanation for these observed effects.* "[40] This concession is important because it tends to shift the debate from whether these events happen to how they take place. Still, Hyman and many of his skeptical colleagues are unwilling to admit that these phenomena are real. He states, "Inexplicable statistical departures from chance, however, are a far cry from compelling evidence for anomalous cognition"[41]–and, presumably, intercessory prayer. This response seems capricious and arbitrary in the extreme, and suggests a double standard. Which statistics are acceptable and which are not? Can we pick and choose? If one denies the validity of the statistical approach in parapsychology or prayer, how can one defend its use in other controversial areas of science?

EMERGING THEORIES

For several years the favorite charge of critics has been that evidence for intercessory prayer and distant mental effects does not exist. But as the experimental evidence has increased and its quality improved, they now seem to be resurrecting an old complaint–that, as we've seen, there is no accepted scientific theory to explain these phenomena. This charge ignores significant developments within science that lend theoretical support to the events we have been examining, including intercessory prayer.

The model of consciousness that is needed to accommodate distant mental intentions is one which, in my opinion, recognizes a nonlocal quality of the mind. "Nonlocal mind" is a term I introduced in 1989 in my book Recovering the Soul.[42] According to this concept, consciousness cannot be completely localized or confined to specific points in space, such as brains or bodies, or to discrete points in time, such as the present moment. Several models of consciousness have recently been proposed by eminent scientists that embody this quality of the mind. For example:

- David J. Chalmers, a mathematician and cognitive scientist from the University of California at Santa Cruz, has suggested that consciousness is fundamental in the universe, perhaps on a par with matter and energy. It is not derived from anything else, and cannot be reduced to anything more basic.[43,44] His view frees consciousness from its local confinement to the brain, and opens the door for nonlocal, consciousness-mediated events such as we've discussed.
- Physicist Amit Goswami of the University of Oregon's Institute of Theoretical Science has proposed his Science Within Consciousness (SWC) theory, in which consciousness is recognized as a fundamental, causal factor in the universe, not confined to the brain, body, or the present.[45,46]
- Physicist Nick Herbert has long proposed a similar view. He suggests that consciousness abounds in the universe and that we have seriously underestimated the "amount" of it, just as early physicists drastically underestimated the size of the universe.[47,48]
- Nobel physicist Brian D. Josephson, of Cambridge University's Cavendish Laboratory, has proposed that consciousness makes possible "the biological utilization of quantum nonlocality." He believes that nonlocal events exist not only at the subatomic level, but, through the actions of the mind, can be

amplified and emerge in our everyday experience as distant mental events of a broad variety.[49]

- Rupert Sheldrake, the British botanist, has proposed a nonlocal picture of consciousness in his widely known "hypothesis of formative causation."[50,51] Sheldrake sees great promise in his model for distant, mental events such as intercessory prayer.

- Systems theorist Ervin Laszlo has proposed that nonlocal, consciousness-mediated events such as intercessory prayer, telepathy, precognition, and clairvoyance may be explainable through developments in physics concerning the quantum vacuum and zero-point field.[52]

- The late physicist David Bohm proposed that consciousness is present to some degree in everything. "Everything material is also mental and everything mental is also material," he states. "The separation of the two—matter and spirit—is an abstraction. The ground is also one."[53] Bohm's views, like the above hypotheses, liberate consciousness from its confinement to the body and make possible, in principle, the distant, nonlocal phenomena we've examined.

- Robert G. Jahn, former dean of engineering at Princeton University, and his colleagues at the Princeton Engineering Anomalies Research lab, have proposed a model of the mind in which consciousness acts freely through space and time to create actual change in the physical world. Their hypothesis is based on their experimental evidence, which is the largest database ever assembled of the effects of distant intentionality.[54]

- Mathematician C. J. S. Clarke, of the University of Southampton's Faculty of Mathematical Studies, has proposed that "it is necessary to place mind first as the key aspect of the universe." Clarke's hypothesis is based in a quantum logic approach to physics, and takes nonlocality as its starting point.[55]

Although these views are recent, they are part of a long tradition within science. Many of the greatest scientists of this century have been cordial to an extended, unitary model of the mind that permits the sort of distant mental intentions we've been examining.[56] This shows that a nonlocal view of consciousness is not a fringe or radical idea, as critics often claim. Examples include the following:

- Erwin Schrödinger, the Nobel physicist whose wave equations lie at the heart of modern quantum physics: "Mind by its very nature is a singular tantum. I should say: the overall number of minds is just one."[57]
- Sir Arthur Eddington, the eminent astronomer-physicist: "The idea of a universal Mind or Logos would be, I think, a fairly plausible inference from the present state of scientific theory; at least it is in harmony with it."[58]
- Sir James Jeans, the British mathematician, astronomer, and physicist: "When we view ourselves in space and time, our consciousnesses are obviously the separate individuals of a particle-picture, but when we pass beyond space and time, they may perhaps form ingredients of a single continuous stream of life. As it is with light and electricity, so it may be with life; the phenomena may be individuals carrying on separate existences in space and time, while in the deeper reality beyond space and time we may all be members of one body."[59]

SOME CAUTIONS

Many of the above theories rely on developments and interpretations within quantum physics. But let us bear in mind that physics—quantum or otherwise—does not "explain consciousness" or "prove prayer." "Quantum" has recently been applied to everything from psychology to healing to golf. No doubt we shall soon hear about "quantum prayer."

There is not now, nor has there ever been, a consensus among physicists—or scientists in general—about the nature of consciousness. Some respected researchers in the field of neurophysiology, such as William H. Calvin, doubt whether or not physics can contribute anything to understanding consciousness. He asserts, "Consciousness, in any of its varied connotations, certainly isn't located down in the . . . sub-basement of physics. . . . [These] consciousness physicists use mathematical concepts to dazzle rather than enlighten. . . . Such theorists usually avoid the word 'spirit' and say something about quantum fields. . . . All that the consciousness physicists have accomplished is the replacement of one mystery by another."[60]

Some prominent physicists are dubious about how much their field can contribute to our understanding of spirituality. For example, the late John S. Bell, whose famous theorem has generated immense interest in quantum nonlocality, said, "In my opinion, physics has not progressed far enough to link up with psychology or theology or sociology. . . . I don't think Bell's theorem moves you nearer to God."[61]

But when viewed in the context of the growing research in intercessory prayer, perhaps this point of view is too conservative. In the opinion of an increasing number of scientists, physics opens an important window to those interested in distant intentionality and prayer. At a minimum, physics grants us permission, as it were, to entertain the possibility that consciousness may manifest nonlocally in the world. Why? Physics now recognizes the existence of quantum-scale events that are decidedly nonlocal, such as spin correlations between distant subatomic particles. These events share three salient characteristics. They are said to be immediate–i.e., they occur simultaneously; they are unmediated–i.e., they do not depend on any known form of energy for their "transmission"; and they are unmitigated–i.e., their strength does not diminish with increasing spatial separation.[62] Distant, intercessory prayer bears a strong resemblance to these events. Therefore, if physicists have discovered the existence of nonlocal events in the subatomic domain, we are fully justified in exploring our macroscopic world for evidence of nonlocal events as well, such as distant, intercessory prayer. The importance of this contribution from physics is monumental, for it helps legitimize the debate about "mental action at a distance" and intercessory prayer, which has been essentially closed within science for three centuries.

Another caution: Let us recognize that controlled experiments test only one aspect of prayer and are therefore exceedingly limited. To quote British physicist Russell Stannard once more, "Prayer in its totality is multifaceted consisting as it does of worship, thanksgiving, contrition, self-dedication, contemplation, meditation, etc. Intercession is but one component. Not only that, the experiment is

concerned solely with those intercessory prayers offered up on behalf of strangers. Like many others, I suspect that the central core of
intercessory prayer has more to do with the agonizing, involved
prayers of loved ones and intimate friends . . . than with those of
distant strangers."[63]

But let us not be too modest in assessing our harvest. As physician Daniel J. Benor states in a summary of the current status of this
field, *"There are a sufficient number of well-designed, well-
executed studies demonstrating statistically significant effects to
support an assertion that healing is a potent intervention."*[64]

A LOOK TO THE FUTURE

Although we need more experimental data (scientists in every
field say this), the major obstacle in taking intercessory prayer
seriously is not, I think, a lack of empirical evidence. Our major
difficulty is that we seem to be suffering from a failure of the
imagination. Unable to see how prayer could work, too many
people insist that it can not work. Unless we learn to see the world
in new ways, we shall remain unable to engage the evidence for
intercessory prayer that already exists, and we shall be tempted to
dismiss future evidence no matter how strong it proves to be. Physi-
cian-researcher Jan Ehrenwald, writing in *The Journal of Nervous
and Mental Disease,* describes what we are up against:

> It is paradoxical that more than one-half century after the
> advent of relativistic physics and the formulation of quantum
> mechanics, current theories of personality are still steeped in
> the classical Judeo-Christian, Aristotelian, or Cartesian tradi-
> tion. Our neurophysiological models of the organism, our psy-
> chological and psychoanalytic concepts about the "mind," are
> located in Euclidean space and conform to essentially mecha-
> nistic, Newtonian, causal-reductive principles.
>
> What are the hallmarks of the classical model? It conceives
> of personality as a closed, self-contained, homeostatic system
> operating in a universe extended in prerelativistic space and
> time and subject to the ironclad laws of cause and effect. It
> found its classical pictorial representation in Leonardo da Vin-

ci's figure of a male of ideal proportions, safely anchored in the double enclosure of the circle and the square, setting him apart from the rest of the world.[65]

Even those who believe in intercessory prayer generally seem wedded to the classical images to which Ehrenwald refers, which seem hopelessly flawed.[66] They generally conceive of prayer as some sort of energetic signal that is sent up and out to the Almighty, who functions as a kind of satellite relay station who passes on the effect to the recipient of the prayer. There is no evidence whatever in studies of prayer and distant intentionality that these images apply. Still, the cherished hope of many seems to be that some sort of "subtle energy" will one day be detected to explain the distant effects of prayer. Although this conceivably could happen, current evidence suggests that the old energy-based, classical concepts will remain unable to explain the workings of intercessory prayer, and new images will be necessary.[67,68]

Until adequate scientific explanations of intercessory prayer arrive, we need not suspend our belief in prayer nor deny the evidence for it. Even when future explanations are in place, "God does it!" will remain a perfectly reasonable alternative, because any new theory is certain to raise more questions than it will answer, and it is impossible in principle for any scientific theory to disprove the existence and workings of the Absolute.

Another major obstacle to engaging the evidence for intercessory prayer is fear.[69] The instant we acknowledge the data that we can affect living systems positively at a distance through prayer, the possibility is raised that we may be able to harm them as well. This consideration prompts almost everybody to run for cover, including believers in prayer–because, as philosopher Alan Watts once put it, we want to keep God's skirts clean. It is going to be difficult to do so. Several studies in distant intentionality using bacteria and fungi strongly suggest that we can not only increase their growth rates but inhibit them as well.[70,71,72] This prospect should not horrify us. Sometimes we need prayer to be injurious–as when we pray for a cancer to be destroyed, for an obstruction in a coronary artery to be obliterated, or for AIDS viruses to be killed. The negative side of prayer is discussed extensively in my book *Be Careful What You Pray For.*[73]

PRAYER DOES NOT REQUIRE SCIENCE

Although we have focused on the experimental evidence for intercessory prayer, let us recall that prayer does not require science to validate it. There is no need to hold our breath in anticipation of the results of the next double-blind study on prayer. *People test prayer in their individual lives, and one's life is the most important laboratory of all.* However, self-deception is possible, and science is an effective safeguard against some forms of illusion. In our culture, science has undeniably become a potent arbiter of how we construct our world view and how we live our lives. Therefore, if science says something positive about prayer, even those who already believe in prayer may feel empowered in their convictions.

THE RESPIRITUALIZATION OF MEDICINE

The studies in intercessory prayer and distant intentionality represent a major opportunity for a genuine dialogue between medicine and spirituality. This debate needs desperately to go forward.

Modern medicine has become one of the most spiritually malnourished professions in our society. Because medicine has so thoroughly disowned the spiritual component to healing, most healers throughout history would view the profession today as inherently perverse. They would be aghast at how it has squeezed the life juices and the heart out of its calling. Physicians have spiritual needs like anyone else, and they have paid a painful price for ignoring them. It simply does not feel good to practice medicine as if the only thing that matters is the physical; something feels left out and incomplete.

André Malraux, the late French novelist and minister of culture of France, said that the twenty-first century will be spiritual or it will not be at all. I often feel the same way about medicine. It will be respiritualized, or it may not be at all, or at least not in any form we would desire. Yet there is great hope, and the scientific research into the healing effects of prayer, empathy, and love bode well to assist the process of the respiritualization of medicine.

The dangers in the prayer-and-science dialogue are quite real, and we have to navigate these waters carefully. But if we do so–and I am convinced we can–medicine may once again deserve to be called the healing profession.

What role will pastoral caregivers have in this process of infusing the science of medicine with this new sense of spirituality? I am unable to answer that question. Only you as the spiritual representatives within the medical system can answer it. What I do know is that scientific findings are increasingly supporting the importance of spirituality and prayer. Your first challenge may be to take these scientific results seriously and craft your own response to them.

REFERENCES

1. Larry Dossey. *Healing Words* (San Francisco: Harper SanFrancisco, 1993).
2. Daniel J. Benor. *Healing Research*, vols. 1-4 (Munich: Helix Verlag, 1993).
3. Donald Evans. *Spirituality and Human Nature* (Albany, New York: SUNY Press, 1993).
4. Brian Inglis. *Natural and Supernatural: A History of the Paranormal* (Bridport, Dorset, England: Prism Press, 1992), 43-112.
5. *The Journal of Religion and Psychical Research* is published by The Academy of Religion and Physical Research, P.O.B. 614, Bloomfield, CT 06002.
6. *The Christian Parapsychologist* is published by The Churches' Fellowship for Psychical and Spiritual Studies, South Road, North Somercotes, North Louth, Lincolnshire LN11 7PT, England.
7. Michael Stoeber and Hugo Meynell (eds). *Critical Reflections on the Paranormal* (Albany: SUNY Press, 1996).
8. Erlendur Haraldsson and Thorstein Thorsteinsson. "Psychokinetic effects on yeast: An exploration experiment." In: W. E. Roll, R. L. Morris, J. D. Morris (Eds.) *Research in Parapsychology 1972.* (Metuchen, NJ: Scarecrow Press 1973), 20-21. See also: Erlendur Haraldsson. "Research on alternative medicine in Iceland," MISAHA Newsletter (Monterey Institute for the Study of Alternative Healing Arts), April-June, 1995, 3-5.
9. William G. Braud. "Human interconnectedness: Research indications." *ReVision* 1992;14(3):140-8. See also: D. Radin and R. Nelson. "Consciousness-related effects in random physical systems." *Foundations of Physics* 1989; 19: 1499-1514.
10. Robert G. Jahn. "Report on the academy of consciousness studies." *Journal of Scientific Exploration* 1995; 9(3): 393-403. See also: Larry Dossey. "What's love got to do with it?" *Alternative Therapies* 1996; 2(3):8-15.
11. Randolph C. Byrd. "Positive therapeutic effects of intercessory prayer in a coronary care unit population." *Southern Medical Journal* 1988; 81:826-29.
12. Keith Stewart Thomson. "The revival of experiments on prayer," *American Scientist* 1996; 84:532-4.
13. William G. Braud. "Conscious interactions with remote biological systems: Anomalous intentionality effects." *Subtle Energies* 1991; 2(1):1-40.

14. Daniel J. Benor. *Healing Research,* vols. 1-4. Munich: Helix Verlag, 1993.

15. Susan J. Armstrong. "Souls in process: A theoretical inquiry into animal psi." In: Michael Stoeber and Hugo Meynell, (eds). *Critical Reflections on the Paranormal* (Albany: SUNY Press, 1996), 133-58.

16. Larry Dossey. "Four-legged forms of prayer" and "A [veterinarian] doctor tests prayer." In: *Prayer Is Good Medicine* (San Francisco: HarperSanFrancisco, 1996), 112-23.

17. E. Haraldsson and T. Thorsteinsson. "Psychokinetic effects on yeast: An exploratory experiment." In: W.C. Roll, R.L. Morris, J.D. Morris, (eds.) *Research in Parapsychology 1972* (Metuchen, NJ: Scarecrow Press, 1973), 20-21.

18. For a glimpse into life of this remarkable woman and her talented husband, see Ambrose A. and Olga N. Worrall, *Explore Your Psychic World.* Memorial edition. (Columbus, OH: Ariel Press, 1989. First published by: New York: Harper and Row, 1970).

19. Beverly Rubik and Elizabeth Rauscher. "Effects on motility behavior and growth rate of *Salmonella typhimurium* in the presence of Olga Worrall." In: W.G. Roll (ed.), *Research in Parapsychology 1979* (Metuchen, NJ: Scarcrow Press, 1980) 140-42. Also: E. Rauscher. "Human volitional effects on a model bacterial system." *Subtle Energies* 1990; 1(1):21-41

20. Randolph C. Byrd. "Positive therapeutic effects of intercessory prayer in a coronary care unit population." *Southern Medical Journal* 1988; 81:826-29.

21. Larry Dossey. "Prayer in the coronary care unit." *Healing Words* (San Francisco: HarperSanFrancisco, 1993), 179-86.

22. Russell Stannard. Communication to Canon Michael Perry, Sub-Dean of Durham Cathedral, Durham, England, April 1997.

23. Jean Kinkead Martine. "Working for a living." *Parabola* 1996; XXI:4,50-4.

24. Jean Kinkead Martine. *ibid.*, p. 50.

25. Larry Dossey. *Healing Words* (San Francisco: HarperSanFrancisco, 1993), 23-28.

26. Catherine Osgerby. "Scientists put intercession to the test," *Church Times* (England), 18 April, 1997.

27. G.R. Price. "Science and the supernatural." *Science* 1955; 122:359-67.

28. Hermann von Helmholtz. Quoted in: Michael Murphy, *The Future of the Body* (Los Angeles: Jeremy Tarcher, 1992), 345.

29. Editorial, "Scanning the issue," in *Proceedings of the IEEE.* March 1976; LXIV(3):291. Cited in: Russell Targ and Harold Puthoff, *Mind-Reach* (New York: Delta, 1977), 169.

30. G.R. Price, 360.

31. Gerald Feinberg. "Precognition—a memory of things future." In: L. Oteri (Ed.). *Quantum Physics and Parapsychology.* (New York: Parapsychology Foundation) 1975:54-73.

32. Meehl PE, Scriven M. Compatibility of science and ESP. *Science* 1956; 123:14-5.

33. Jeffrey S. Levin. "How prayer heals: A theoretical model." *Alternative Therapies* 1996; 2(1):66-73.

34. Fielding H. Garrison. *History of Medicine,* Fourth Edition (Philadelphia: W.B. Saunders, 1929), 435-7.

35. Eugene Mills. "Giving up on the hard problem." *Journal of Consciousness Studies* 1966; 3(1):26-32.

36. Larry Dossey. "Response to Gracely." *Alternative Therapies* 1995; 1(5):104-8.

37. Larry Dossey. "How good is the evidence? Prayer, mediation, and parapsychology." *Healing Words* (San Francisco: HarperSanFrancisco, 1993), 243-7.

38. David J. Hufford. "Cultural and social perspectives on alternative medicine: background and assumptions." *Alternative Therapies* 1995; 1(1):53-61.

39. B.R. Cassileth, E.J. Lusk, T.B. Strouse, F.J. Bodenheimer. "Contemporary unorthodox treatments in cancer medicine: a study of patients, treatments, and practitioners." *Annals of Internal Medicine* 1984; 10:105-12.

40. Hyman R. "Evaluation of a program on anomalous mental phenomena." *Journal of Scientific Exploration* 1995; 10(1):31-58.

41. Hyman R. *ibid.,* 43.

42. Larry Dossey. *Recovering the Soul* (New York: Bantam, 1989).

43. David J. Chalmers. "The puzzle of conscious experience," *Scientific American* 1995; 273(6):80-6.

44. David J. Chalmers. *The Conscious Mind* (New York: Oxford University Press, 1996).

45. Amit Goswami. *The Self-Aware Universe: How Consciousness Creates the Material World* (New York: Tarcher/Putnam, 1993).

46. Amit Goswami. "Science within consciousness: A progress report." Talk delivered at a seminar on consciousness, University of Lisbon, Lisbon, Portugal, 1996.

47. Nick Herbert. *Quantum Reality* (New York: Dation, 1986).

48. Nick Herbert. *Elemental Mind* (New York: Dation, 1993).

49. Brian D. Josephson and F. Pallikara-Viras. "Biological utilization of quantum nonlocality." *Foundations of Physics* 1991; 21:197-207.

50. Rupert Sheldrake. *A New Science of Life.* (Los Angeles: Tarcher, 1981).

51. Rupert Sheldrake. *The Presence of the Past* (New York: Times Books, 1988).

52. Ervin Laszlo. *The Interconnected Universe: Conceptual Foundations of Transdisciplinary Unified Theory* (River Edge, NJ:World Scientific Publishing Co., 1995).

53. David Bohm quoted in Renée Weber. *Dialogue with Scientists and Sages: The Search for Unity* (London: Arkana, 1990), 101 and 151.

54. Robert G. Jahn and Brenda J. Dunne. *Margins of Reality: The Role of Consciousness in the Physical World* (New York: Harcourt Brace Jovanovich, 1987).

55. C.J.S. Clarke. "The nonlocality of mind," *Journal of Consciousness Studies* 1995; 2(3):231-40.

56. Ken Wilber (ed). *Quantum Questions: The Mystical Writings of the World's Great Physicists* (Boston: Shambhala, 1984).

57. Erwin Schrödinger. *What is Life? and Mind and Matter* (London: Cambridge University Press, 1969),145.

58. Arthur Eddington. "Defense of Mysticism." In: Ken Wilber (ed). *Quantum Questions: The Mystical Writings of the World's Great Physicists.* (Boston: Shambhala, 1984), 206.

59. James Jeans. *Physics and Philosophy* (New York: Dover, 1981), 204.

60. William H. Calvin. *How Brains Think: Evolving Intelligence, Then and Now.* (New York: Basic Books, 1996). Quotations from "Mechanisms of the Soul," Review of Calvin's *How Brains Think* by Marcia Bartusiak, New York Times Book Review, 29 December, 1996.

61. John S. Bell. Interview. OMNI, May 1988, 85 ff.

62. Nick Herbert. *Quantum Reality* (New York: Dation, 1986), 214.

63. Russell Stannard. Communication to Canon Michael Perry, Sub-Dean of Durham Cathedral, Durham, England, April 1997.

64. Daniel J. Benor. "'Healing' in Great Britain." *Advances* 1996; 12(4):75-7.

65. Jan Ehrenwald. "A neurophysiological model of psi phenomena," *Journal of Nervous and Mental Disease* 1972: 154(6):406-18.

66. Larry Dossey. "Models of prayer." In: *Healing Words* (San Francisco: HarperSanFrancisco, 1993), 8.

67. Larry Dossey. "But is it energy? Reflections on consciousness, healing, and the new paradigm." *Subtle Energies* 1992; 3(3):69-82.

68. Larry Dossey. "Healing, energy, and consciousness: Into the future or a retreat into the past?" *Subtle Energies* 1994; 5(1):1-33.

69. Larry Dossey. "Running scared: how we hide from who we are." *Alternative Therapies* 1997; 3(2):8-15.

70. Barry J. "General and comparative study of the psychokinetic effect on a fungus culture." *Journal of Parapsychology* 1968; 32:237-43.

71. Tedder W, Monty M. "Exploration of long-distance PK: a conceptual replication of the influence of a biological system." In: Roll WG, et al., (eds). *Research in Parapsychology 1980.* (Metuchen, NJ: Scarecrow Press; 1981) 90-93.

72. Nash CB. "Psychokinetic control of bacterial growth." *Journal of the American Society for Psychical Research* 1982; 51:217-21.

73. Larry Dossey. *Be Careful What You Pray For* (San Francisco: HarperSanFrancisco, 1997).

RESPONDENTS

The Laboratory of Religious Experience: A Response to Larry Dossey

John T. VanderZee, DMin, BCC

A friend and former employee of the hospital where I work was recently admitted with a serious exacerbation of a chronic lung ailment. Although he has had many hospitalizations this was the sickest I had ever seen him. Struggling for every breath, he could hardly speak, and his fingers were beginning to turn purple. His two daughters were at his bedside. Trying unsuccessfully to conceal their fear and concern, they asked me to pray for him. My friend could only nod his concurrence. After a period of silence I prayed that the Spirit of God bring calm and peace with each new breath he took.

John T. VanderZee is affiliated with Bloomington Hospital, Bloomington, IN 47402.

[Haworth co-indexing entry note]: "The Laboratory of Religious Experience: A Response to Larry Dossey." VanderZee, John T. Co-published simultaneously in *Journal of Health Care Chaplaincy* (The Haworth Pastoral Press, an imprint of The Haworth Press, Inc.) Vol. 7, No. 1/2, 1998, pp. 39-43; and: *Scientific and Pastoral Perspectives on Intercessory Prayer: An Exchange Between Larry Dossey, M.D. and Health Care Chaplains* (ed: Larry VandeCreek) The Haworth Pastoral Press, an imprint of The Haworth Press, Inc., 1998, pp. 39-43; and: *Scientific and Pastoral Perspectives on Intercessory Prayer: An Exchange Between Larry Dossey, M.D. and Health Care Chaplains* (ed: Larry VandeCreek) Harrington Park Press, an imprint of The Haworth Press, Inc., 1998, pp. 39-43. Single or multiple copies of this article are available for a fee from The Haworth Document Delivery Service [1-800-342-9678, 9:00 a.m. - 5:00 p.m. (EST). E-mail address: getinfo@haworth.com].

39

A scant 30 hours later I came into the patient's room and found him sitting on the edge of his bed and eating dinner. He greeted me enthusiastically while his wife and daughter beamed with delight. *"It was your prayer that did it, chaplain," his daughter said. "Within a few hours after you left, Dad's breathing calmed down and he got a good night's sleep."*

I mumbled something about this being God's doing and that I was a mere instrument, while a flood of contradictory feelings washed over me. I felt embarrassed and heroic, bemused and justified. I remember thinking how naive and childish was her conception of prayer, and how typical of so many people who regard answered prayer primarily in terms of prompt responses to precise requests. The incident spurred me to think more deliberately about my own attitudes regarding prayer, and its role in pastoral care.

Similarly, Dossey has raised some very important questions about how and why hospital chaplains engage patients and families in intercessory prayer. Is prayer a pastoral function which the chaplain feels "an obligation" to discharge, or "a purely religious performance in response to expectations?" Is prayer an activity that can truly effect healing, and might even be valued in partnership with medical intervention?

Dr. Dossey correctly challenges us in health care ministry to "take prayer seriously," because more and more people are doing just that. The field of pastoral care is slowly shifting partly in response to the current captivation with spirituality in our culture. *"Spiritual care" is beginning to replace "pastoral care" as the substance of what we chaplains do, and prayer seems to be viewed increasingly as our central function.*

I wholeheartedly agree with Dr. Dossey that not only prayer in general but intercessory prayer in particular is a vitally important activity for the pastoral care giver. Kenneth Leech rightly maintains that "we are seeking to be ministers of healing and reconciliation through the power of God which is released through the prayer of intercession."[1] While God certainly has the wherewithal to heal and reconcile in the absence of our prayer, we presume that God is also content to heal in response to or in concert with our entreaties on behalf of others. Intercession, so understood, "is a literal standing between, an act of reconciliation, . . . a priestly work in which Christ allows us to share."[1]

Dr. Dossey calls us back to a position of integrity and intentionality regarding intercessory prayer. Unfortunately, he asks us to do it, I think, for the wrong reason. He asks us to take prayer seriously not because it is still the most effective means to convey to hurting people the healing presence of God, but "because of what science is discovering" about prayer.

Now that spirituality is chic and prayer in its varied forms is gaining acceptance, it should not surprise us that the efficacy of prayer has now become a growing focus of scientific experimentation. Dr. Dossey endeavors to show us how this is a good thing, and why we should be eternally grateful to science for finally providing us with the proof of what we had long begun to doubt if not deny.

I have the same discomfort with Dr. Dossey taking such pains to show scientifically that "prayer works" as I do with the highway billboards that smugly splash the same message. Do we want to encourage people to pray because we think they will get what they pray for a good part of the time? Or do we believe prayer is good and even healthful because prayer is communion with God, and God desires the fullness of life and health for us? *Dr. Dossey appears to be less interested in prayer as a way of coming to know and be known by God, and more in prayer as a potent, under-utilized change agent.*

Occasionally it is worthwhile to ponder the wise old adage, "be careful what you pray for, you might just get it." But a rephrasing may be even more prudent: "Be careful that you recognize in faith the answer to prayer when and if it comes." A critical question raised by prayer efficacy research is how can we be sure of what an answer to prayer is if we were to stumble upon it? And if it were possible to know whether or not prayers are answered, is it really science that we should rely on to make that determination?

George Buttrick in his classic work, *Prayer* argues that science is an inadequate evaluator of prayer because its purview is "too external, too fractional . . . and too analytical."[2] Science, by definition, is forced to examine prayer solely within the framework imposed by natural law. Even the contribution of quantum physics greatly extends but does not transcend the bounds of natural law. Science is a poor judge of the efficacy of intercessory prayer because it is not very good at addressing the nuances of human intent. Moreover it is altogether disinterested in the whole question of divine disclosure. *There is no better determinant of prayer's capability than the lived-out existence of the pray-er.*

Measuring prayer's ability to increase the rate of growth of micro-organisms in test tubes, or lessen the need that a patient might have for post-operative pain medication may spark curiosity. But there are other important things that prayer produces which are much more difficult to measure. We might well contemplate with Edward Bauman, "who can see the effects of the love made available when one person prays for another? Who can measure the courage that flows into a tired heart when prayer is offered for a loved one? Who can isolate all the forces in the new situation created by earnest and fervent intercession among friends?"[3]

Nevertheless, I felt myself cheering Dr. Dossey on as he evoked quantum physics in his defense of the supernatural effects of prayer. As science makes more and more discoveries, it also recognizes the vastness of the horizon of knowledge still to be touched. Prayer may be one such under-explored realm. As enticing as this may be to consider, I am not convinced that we in pastoral ministry have a significant role to play here.

This is not to say that there is nothing about prayer that merits scientific study. We have much to learn, it seems to me, about how and why and in what manner people pray in times of physical extremity or personal crisis. It would be fascinating to explore what answered or unanswered prayer means to different people. What might be learned from examining the prayer life of physicians or other health care professionals? How do the prayers of believing chronically ill people evolve as their disease progresses? Still, we need to be very careful about the conclusions and judgements at which we arrive from such studies.

Dr. Dossey invites us to contribute mightily to the healing endeavor by praying for patients because there is growing scientific proof of prayer's effectiveness. For the person of faith, however, communion with God has its own sufficient rewards. The real miracle of intercessory prayer is when the reality of God's grace and love is quickened in someone through the ministry of another. The transformed heart is the kind of healing that surpasses any material benefits that medical science could possibly measure. What Edward W. Bauman wrote almost 40 years ago rings true also today:

> Up to the present time, the final and conclusive proof of prayer remains within the field of individual religious experience. We know that God answers prayer only when God makes [God's self] known . . . and responds only when we are sure of [God's] response in our own lives.[3]

REFERENCES

1. Kenneth Leech. *True Prayer: An Invitation to Christian Spirituality* (San Francisco: Harper and Row, 1980), 164.

2. George A. Buttrick. *Intercessory Prayer* (Nashville: Abingdon-Cokesbury Press, 1942), 85-86.

3. Edward W. Bauman. *Intercessory Prayer* (Philadelphia: The Westminster Press, 1958), 31.

Response to Larry Dossey

Marsha Cutting, MDiv, BCC

I have not had the option of not believing in intercessory prayer for many years. When I returned to the church in my mid-twenties, it became clear to me that if nothing else, prayer changed the one who prayed, made her more aware of the needs of others and more open to possible ways of being useful. Then, while serving a small rural parish, I called upon a man who was hospitalized in a large teaching hospital. He and his wife were the parents of a parishioner. He had gone to his doctor with sores on his toes; his wife reported that he had been given ointment and sent home. When the pain from the sores became unbearable, he presented to the Emergency Department, where his diabetes was diagnosed and treatment for gangrene was initiated. Parts of one foot and then the other were amputated. Then one leg was taken off below the knee. This appeared to be more than his body was able to tolerate; doctors wanted to remove the other leg, but it was felt he was too ill to tolerate the operation. I visited him and his wife in the Intensive Care Unit, where he lay unresponsive to the world around him. His wife told me, outside the room, that the doctors had told her that he almost certainly would die, that only a miracle would save him. So we

---

Marsha Cutting is affiliated with the Department of Pastoral Care, Capital District Psychiatric Center, Albany, NY 12208.

[Haworth co-indexing entry note]: "Response to Larry Dossey." Cutting, Marsha. Co-published simultaneously in *Journal of Health Care Chaplaincy* (The Haworth Pastoral Press, an imprint of The Haworth Press, Inc.) Vol. 7, No. 1/2, 1998, pp. 45-61; and: *Scientific and Pastoral Perspectives on Intercessory Prayer: An Exchange Between Larry Dossey, M.D. and Health Care Chaplains* (ed: Larry VandeCreek) The Haworth Pastoral Press, an imprint of The Haworth Press, Inc., 1998, pp. 45-61; and: *Scientific and Pastoral Perspectives on Intercessory Prayer: An Exchange Between Larry Dossey, M.D. and Health Care Chaplains* (ed: Larry VandeCreek) Harrington Park Press, an imprint of The Haworth Press, Inc., 1998, pp. 45-61. Single or multiple copies of this article are available for a fee from The Haworth Document Delivery Service [1-800-342-9678, 9:00 a.m. - 5:00 p.m. (EST). E-mail address: getinfo@haworth.com].

prayed for a miracle. In the weeks that followed, I suspect we both had moments when we wondered if death wouldn't have been kinder, but six months later, he walked into church for his eldest granddaughter's wedding on two prosthetic legs. As Larry Dossey notes, *"People test prayer in their individual lives; and one's life is the most important laboratory of all." Disbelief, for me, is not an option; curiosity certainly is.* One of my frustrations with the paper by Dossey is that his questions are not necessarily mine. I don't have problems with prayer in laboratories or prayer for other life forms, for example; all are a part of God's creation. *I also have my own questions which Dossey does not address. In addition to the questions of the scientist about whether intercessory prayer "works," there is another set of questions raised by the theologian. After all, people who believe that a man who died nearly 2000 years ago can be present with us when we gather around a table which holds bread and wine really shouldn't have trouble with the idea that intercessory prayer could affect medical conditions.* The theological questions include those about God's omniscience (do we need to tell God someone is in need of healing?), God's beneficence (does God need our appeals to act favorably in someone's behalf?), God's intentionality (why would God heal one person who was prayed for and not another?) and the relative merit of the intentions (should prayer determine the outcome of the championship basketball game for my school's team?). I will return to these after I discuss some of the issues Dossey raises.

The question of "testing" God deserves more serious consideration than Dossey gives it. There is, of course, a Biblical injunction against testing God (Deut. 6:16) which Jesus quotes while he is himself being tested following his baptism. The injunction has its origins in Ex. 17:7. The Hebrews have been delivered from the Egyptian captivity and are wandering in the desert. They are finding the transition from slavery to independence a challenging one; they mentally gaze back at the fleshpots of Egypt with vision blurred by the desert's dust and heat. God has provided manna and quails, but now water appears to be lacking. The people find fault with Moses, who reframes their obstreperousness as "test(ing) the Lord" (Ex. 17:2). After water is provided, with God's intervention, Moses indicates that they "tested the Lord, saying, 'Is the Lord among us or not?'" (Ex. 17:7). This question has not previously been raised, a fact which Rabbinic commentators have not missed. The eminent Israeli Biblical scholar Nahama Leibowitz quotes Rabbi Isaac Abravanel (Spain, 1437-1508) as defending the Hebrews thusly:

> If they lacked drinking water, then they were justified in complaining. To whom should they have turned if not to their leader Moses, to perform some wonder? Why should this conduct of theirs be termed: 'trying?' It was surely an absolutely legitimate and essential request![1]

She then cites other Rabbinic scholars who argue that the fault of the Israelites lay in making their loyalty to God conditional. One argument is that they wish to see God perform miracles for them in exchange for their worship; another is that they make their worship contingent on a display of God's mercy toward them. Leibowitz says, "The sin of trying to find out whether belief in God was worthwhile, was the one with which the Israelites were charged at Massah."[2] She quotes Rabbi Moses Nachmanides (Spain, 1194-1270), who writes, "We are therefore absolutely forbidden to test the Torah or the Prophet. Loyalty to God may not be conditional, dependent on signs and wonders, since it is not his will to perform miracles for any man, at any time . . ."[3]

Do experiments on the efficacy of intercessory prayer violate this prohibition? They could, if they are intended to prove the existence of God, as in the formulation suggested by Keith Stewart Thomson,[4] the "skeptical scientist" to whom Dossey refers. (I'm not sure I want to think about what it means that a scientist has advanced a more carefully considered theological perspective on prayer experiments than many of the reviewers of *Healing Words* published in theological/religious periodicals.)

But the experiment wouldn't necessarily have to be framed as "testing God," and indeed most seem not to be. They can be framed as seeking to understand more about God, God's work in the world and/or our part in God's work. This does not, however, mean that others will not seize upon the results to use as "proof" of God's existence (or nonexistence, as the case may be). In light of the fate which befell Ananias and Sapphira when they "agreed together to put the Spirit of the Lord to the test," (Acts 5:9), one hopes that this might not happen, but things seen, or proved, tend to be more attractive than things not seen or proved. The same Greek word εκπειραζω forms the basis of this tempting, the tempting Jesus refers to, and, in the Septuigent, the Israelites tempting of God. Ananias and Sapphira, of course, have tempted, or tested, God by thinking that God will not know that they are holding back part of the proceeds of their land sale; Kittel and Friedrich note, "What is meant is that the couple, by their conduct, have challenged the Spirit of the Lord, who searches all things (1 C 1:10), whether He would observe the deception."[5] The impertinence of humans testing God is underscored when one realizes that the Greek word εκπειραζω and its Hebrew counterpart used in the Exodus and Deuteronomy passages are most often used in relation to God testing humanity. The scriptures consider it appropriate for the Creator to test the creatures; they do not consider it appropriate for the creatures to test the Creator.

There remains the question of whether the prayer experiments test the God worshipped by Christians and other theists. *It remains open to question whether experiments in "mental intentionality" have anything to do with God.* The department of which I am part works at being open to a wide range of religious perspectives. On the worship table in our chapel are a Torah text, placed there by representatives of the Jewish community; a chalice placed there by a Roman Catholic representative; an incense burner in the shape of the "Om," given by a Hindu staff member; a NRSV Bible provided by the local Council of Churches; a plate of blue corn placed there by representatives of the Native American community; a Qur'an, prayer rug and arrow marking the direction of Qiblah from the Muslims; and a zafu placed by a Buddhist. Being inclusive is important to us, but this inclusivity is built on honoring each of our traditions, not on trying to meld them into one. On Sunday morning, the table is cleared and set for Communion; for the High Holy Days, the shofar, candles and Kiddush cup replace the usual items on the table. Muslims who make their daily prayers use the prayer rug, not the zafu.

The same is true of our prayer traditions. Buddhists, being non-theists, pray differently than Christians, who are theists. Jews and Christians, theists both, pray differently; the expectation of bedside prayer (or in our case, deskside prayer, since patients in our hospital are only rarely in bed during the day, and often seek us out in our offices) comes as something of a shock to the new Jewish chaplain (or so my friends have told me). I found I needed to adjust to the expectation that I would bless religious medals, but in the absence of our Roman Catholic chaplain, currently hospitalized with a spinal cord injury, I do. Most chaplains live in an ecumenical, interfaith world; it is a challenge and a blessing to be grounded in our own traditions and also open to those of others, though I personally find I am most likely to feel that tension with Christians whose theological perspective is markedly different from my own. I certainly would never "inform Buddhists and others who differ from our cultural norms that they aren't really praying," but I might well discuss with them how our understandings of prayer are similar and different, a discussion that can happen only when I am clear about my own tradition.

All of this is to say that for me, as a Christian, while the definition of prayer as "communication with the Absolute" can include my understanding of prayer, I start to have problems with it when I see it played out in Dossey's paper. For me, as a Christian, prayer involves God, who, although within each of us, also exists apart from us. We use a variety of metaphors from God as the "isness" of life (Meister Eckhardt) to God as womb; from God as the underground river of life to God as eagle, and yes, sometimes, God as father. But clearly, for most Christians (and, I suspect for most other theists) God is more than the psychic soup in which we all sink our roots. God has an existence and an intentionality apart from humanity.

In considering definitions, it occurs to me that for the scientist, facts and numbers are significant objects of concern, and for the theologian, words are. So I notice that Dossey uses the word "prayer" and its derivatives in a variety of ways, and sometimes in ways that engender confusion rather than clarity. He offers a definition of prayer as "communication with the Absolute." The discussion and examples which follow, however, call this definition into question. Is "focused attention" communication with the Absolute? It may or may not be. Is "mental intentionality" communication with the Absolute? Perhaps, but not necessarily. Is entering "a sacred, reverential, prayer-like state of mind" the same as prayer? The problem with these various definitions is that they begin to define prayer on the basis of what the person is experiencing, without reference to "the Absolute." This distinction is important. I pray, using centering prayer (as well as other prayer forms). I also have been hypnotized, and can put myself into trance using self-hypnosis. Experientially, these two feel similar, and the people who study brain waves might wish to argue that they are similar. I am clear, however, that they are not the same. What differentiates them is "communication with the Absolute." Psychologist Lawrence LeShan has done extensive work in the area of psi and its relationship to healing, most of it with no reference to "the Absolute," as he makes clear in the final chapter of *The Medium, the Mystic and the Physicist.*[6] After detailing in previous chapters the shifts in consciousness involved in his healing work, he then relates, in "A New Note on a Work in Progress," a dawning appreciation for a dimension of life he refers to as "the All."

These distinctions, and the careful use of language in speaking of prayer, are important because of the impact they have on people's lives. If we blur the distinction about "communication with the Absolute," it becomes easy to think about prayer as something that we do, on our own. Its efficacy then comes to depend on our personal characteristics or on our particular practice, and we begin to move from mystery to magic.

In thinking about this paper, I found that I was captured by the words of the chaplain Dossey quotes, "Look, I need to get something straight. I heard your lecture this morning–and if I understand you correctly, you're claiming that intercessory prayer actually works." I asked a group of chaplains, "Can you see yourself asking that?" Most said no, although several said they could imagine themselves thinking it. One said he could, saying that his questions about intercessory prayer had their genesis at least partly in the uses to which it is put–people praying for their football team to win, etc. But the anonymous chaplain's question has some old roots, and it is important to be aware of them. David J. Hufford, writing about "Epistemologies in Religious Healing,"[7] talks of "centuries of theological development which, following the Reformation and the Enlightenment, moved sharply away from empirical religious claims."[8] He notes the reactions of Reformation theologians to the prevalence of "empirical claims, from mystical visions, to the miracles of saints, and all sorts of prodigious answers to prayer" within Medieval religion and quotes John Cerullo:

> The God described by Reformation thinkers (especially followers of Calvin) simply will not irrupt into either the natural or the social environment as directly or as regularly as does that of Catholicism. The Catholic world was permeated by supernatural manifestations . . . Direct interventions by the heavenly ream were normal, expected (even invocable) . . . Protestantism denied most of them . . . In the final analysis, only one undeniable supernatural event was allotted Protestant man: the devolution of God's sovereign grace.[9]

Jeremy T. Law looks to the events of this century as raising questions about the efficacy of intercessory prayer, noting:

> To ponder the unprecedented scale of its tragedy: the sheer human waste occasioned by the First World War; the Jewish Holocaust of the Second; the nuclear and ecological shadows which are now cast over all humanities activities; the startling inhumanities of the conflicts in Bosnia and Rwanda, is to cast doubt upon the ability of prayer to influence events.[10]

Within the Evangelical community in the United States, according to Leonard Sweet,[11] the efficacy of prayer was a given, although physical healing was seen as a secondary value, and the deepening of religious life and belief as the primary. He notes that for this reason, Evangelicals have not been particularly interested in experiments in prayer. The belief in the efficacy of intercessory prayer, however, was challenged by the coming of the Pentecostal movement in the early part of this century. This was a movement from which Evangelicals wished to distance themselves, and the emphasis on the efficacy of intercessory prayer was sacrificed to this end.

Thomas Furman Hewitt[12] notes that Protestant theologians such as John A.T. Robinson (*Honest to God,* 1963, and *Exploration into God,* 1967), Douglas Rhymes (*Prayer in the Secular City,* 1967), and Paul van Buren (*The Secular Meaning of the Gospel: Based on an Analysis of Its Language,* 1963) questioned God as having a separate existence apart from humanity. This, in turn, led them to question traditional Christian concepts of prayer, and intercessory prayer in particular.

There also are contemporary underpinnings to the anonymous chaplain's words. Bruce Epperly argues that "dysfunctional" understandings of prayer, which operate at a subconscious level, make it difficult for many Christians to take prayer seriously. He writes:

> The primary dysfunctional images of prayer are as follows: (1) An omnipotent God is ultimately responsible for illness, that is, illness is "God's will." (2) Illness is maintained in the traditional versions of *The Book of Common Prayer* as a divine visitation, for the sake of correction, reproof, or punishment. (3) Illness is the result of sin and concomitantly, well-being is a sign of personal goodness and divine favor. (4) Healing is a product of supernatural intervention, grounded solely in God's omnipotent and arbitrary will.[13]

He then offers an understanding of prayer which speaks to these images, as well as many of the other questions Christians have about prayer.

Yet another reason that prayer is the subject of so many questions and doubts is the lack of emphasis it receives in many seminaries, and the consequent lack of confidence felt by many clergy. Carnegie Samuel Calian, president and professor of theology at the Pittsburgh Theological Seminary, writes:

> During seminary years we often subordinate the development of our prayer life for the information and stimulation provided in our courses. We may know that there is no need for division between prayer life and intellectual pursuits; however, when we analyze where we spend most of our time, the classroom and the library often overshadow the chapel.[14]

Daniel Day Lewis suggests that more than a question of time is involved:

> It is well known to theological faculties that students feel a special need for guidance in the private life of devotion and

prayer, and that they rarely feel they are given sufficient help in this matter. Prayer may become more difficult when questions about God have become matters of intellectual analysis, and the inevitable season of theological confusion sets in. Personal problems such as self-doubt may create difficulties in the devotional life. One effect of the years of theological study is, in more cases than we might readily admit, a serious upset of the life of prayer, and in some cases very nearly putting it altogether to one side for a time.[15]

The seminary at which I studied was graced by the presence of the late Henri Nouwen, who taught courses on prayer, among other subjects. These apparently focused on writings about prayer; they did not include prayer itself. (For reasons of scheduling and course distribution, I did not have the opportunity to take one of these courses.) Thus it was that students went to Nouwen and asked him to teach them how to pray. He agreed to do so, and a group of students gathered with him weekly in a small chapel, struggling against the physical demands of sleep-deprived bodies to learn centering prayer. I was fortunate enough to be part of that group, and it was the beginning of an important part of my spiritual journey. But this opportunity was an uncommon one at the time. I have some hope that this is changing; the seminary intern who worked with our department this year tells me that this same seminary now offers spiritual direction for any students who are interested. She didn't tell me (and I didn't ask) how many were.

And finally, there is our experience as chaplains. Working in a state psychiatric hospital, I sometimes find myself in a conference room on one of our units attending a treatment review on Wednesday morning. With a doctor, nurses, a psychologist, a social worker, a nutritionist and a rehabilitation counselor, I use the language of psychiatric caregiving to discuss the strengths and needs of the patient whose treatment is being reviewed.

In the evening, I may be leading a worship service in that same conference room for patients who are restricted to the unit and thus unable to attend the Sunday morning chapel service. I use another type of language, and I have at times been struck by the contrast of these two experiences at different times in the same environment.

And I wonder if the anonymous chaplain could have been responding not only out of doubts about the effects of his prayer, but out of the somewhat unsettling effect of having the usually separate worlds of science and faith brought into juxtaposition.

I suspect that most chaplains are used to having to shift between these two languages on a regular basis, but are not so used to using both together, much less hearing someone else use them simultaneously. Each language employs a model of reality which is only a model, not reality itself. Each may be more or less useful in a given situation. But it is challenging to use both models at the same time. Jungian psychology is not more "real" than self psychology, for example, it is a different way of conceptualizing something. The question is not which is real but which is more useful, which one gives rise to treatment which is helpful to people.

In the course of reflecting on this paper I have to admit I have had uncharitable moments in which I was inclined to think of Larry Dossey as the Jack Kevorkian of prayer: I am glad that someone is raising these issues, but I don't necessarily like the way he's doing it. I wish Dossey's work was more informed by contemporary theological scholarship. I have been frustrated by his simplistic formulations of Christian theology and Biblical interpretation, formulations which then allow him to dismiss consideration of them. I doubt that he would be impressed by someone who wrote an article about a scientific subject based on a popular culture understanding of the subject. I am frustrated by someone who writes an article about a theological subject with apparently scant acquaintance with contemporary scholarship in the field. For example, Dossey writes that those who believe in intercessory prayer "generally conceive of prayer as some sort of energetic signal that is sent up and out to the Almighty, who functions as a kind of satellite relay station who passes on the effect to the recipient of the prayer." None of the numerous authors I consulted in the course of formulating this response offered anything remotely like this. Some, most notably Bruce Epperly, offer an understanding of prayer and of God's action in the world which is quite emphatically outside the "classical model" to which Dossey refers. Epperly argues for an image of God which is "holistic and relational," writing:

Though God is active in the formation of each event, God's own aim for health, healing and beauty is always relational and contextual. It occurs in the midst of the complicated web of life which characterizes the dynamic existence of each being.[16]

Similarly, Dossey reports his conclusion that the most common image of prayer in our culture is something like "talking aloud or to yourself, to a white, male, cosmic parent figure who prefers to be addressed in English." I wonder who his "thousands of Americans" are. Are they people who are connected with faith communities, where images of God have been the subject of vigorous and often heated debate? And are his thousands of Americans capable of addressing God in a language other than English?

There are places in Dossey's paper where it seems that although he has left fundamentalism,[17] fundamentalism may not have left him. I hope he's only teasing us when he writes, "A sanction to pray for microbes can be found in the Lord's Prayer. When we pray for our daily bread, this presumably includes praying for the yeast cells that make it rise," but I'm not sure he is. I know that I certainly have something much less concrete than "asking that the bacteria it (food) contains be put out of commission" in mind when I say grace before meals. And when I read, "If love is crucial to the success of psi experiments, and if 'God is love,' then the Almighty appears to be less nervous than some believers about entering the parapsychology lab," I'm reminded of the old pseudo-syllogism:

God is love,
Love is blind,
Ray Charles is blind,
Ray Charles is God.

The idea of "nonlocality" is not as foreign to Christianity as Dossey seems to think. We see ourselves as a community of believers, those now on earth and those now eternally with God. The Orthodox represent this visually with the gold spheres surrounding the heads of icons. The gold spheres depict the realm of eternity, from which these saints are peering into the world which we inhabit. I am reminded of this by the words of Sir James Jeans which Dossey quotes:

> When we view ourselves in space and time, our conscious-nesses are obviously the separate individuals of a particle-picture, but when we pass beyond space and time, they may perhaps form ingredients of a single continuous stream of life. As it is with light and electricity, so it may be with life; the phenomena may be individuals carrying on separate exis-tences in space and time, while in the deeper reality beyond space and time we may all be members of one body.

This sounds like a parallel to the images we use of the church as the body of Christ and the communion of saints.

In spite of these frustrations with the paper, Dossey's work is useful and important, and too little considered by the religious community, chaplains included. Bernard N. Nathanson[18] reports on "an admittedly cursory survey of the religious bookshops in New York City" in which he found that none of them carried Dossey's writings. It is important for a reason which Dossey offers: ". . . if science says something positive about prayer, even those who already believe in prayer may feel empowered in their convictions." Perhaps we may even be empowered into speech. I pray more than I talk about praying, but both may be important. Patients in the hospital where I work frequently request prayer, most often prayer for a specific need. But staff do so less frequently. How would it be different for staff if they knew that their work was supported by the prayers of the community?

Recently our hospital went through a reconfiguration. This was not a euphemism for layoffs or downsizing, but it was a fairly complete reorganization of the way that the patients and staff were distributed among wards. While many staff members were hopeful about the eventual results, most found the process stressful and had at least some anxiety about the short-term results. During the time for intercessory prayer in the church I attend, I lifted up the staff and patients and mentioned the impending reorganization. A few days later, a staff member mentioned that she had had a call from a former staff member who is a congregant at the church in question. She seemed to appreciate the support from the former staff member, as well as the fact that I had prayed for the staff and patients. F.

Eppling Reincuty, a former president of Southern Seminary, is quoted as saying, "To be a Christian is to have the sense of being prayed for."[19] Because the Catholic chaplain here currently is hospitalized, a Roman Catholic brother has been bringing Communion to our patients. Several have noted his reminder to them that the hosts have been blessed for their use by his community and that his community is holding them in prayer.

And, indeed, we who write these responses are impelled into speaking about what we believe. I don't recall our chaplains' group having discussed prayer prior to my introducing the topic in the course of formulating this response. I agree with Dossey when he writes, "The studies in intercessory prayer and distant intentionality represent a major opportunity for a genuine dialogue between medicine and spirituality." My hope is that the current volume may make a contribution to that dialogue, perhaps beginning to introduce some of the current theological scholarship which I see as lacking thus far.

With that in mind, I want to return to some of the theological questions about intercessory prayer. These include the question asked frequently by patients in this hospital, "Why isn't God answering my prayer?" They also include the questions inherent in the remarks of the doctor treating a patient with Hodgkins Disease who declined a bone marrow transplant and attributed her subsequent recovery to prayer:

> I don't think she was healed by God. I see no rational basis for God to heal Nancy and not others. I've seen too many equally wonderful people succumb to disease and die, people who were just as lovely as Nancy and just as religious and prayed just as hard to get better. But they died in agony. It's hard for me to accept a God who would pick and choose like that.[20]

Also included are the questions mentioned previously about God's omniscience, God's beneficence and the relative merit of intentions.

Law locates petitionary prayer in the tension between the "now" and the "not yet," which is an important way of understanding where we are–out of the garden, not yet to the city of God. The reign of God is inaugurated with the resurrection of the Christ, but it is not yet fully completed. We're called to live into the new reality, to participate in it, even though the old reality may be overwhelmingly present. Law writes:

> All petitionary prayer is, in one degree or another, prayer for the coming kingdom. It is the attempt to see the present, and see it as it actually is, but set against the contours of the promised new creation which has entered the world in an anticipatory way with the resurrection of Christ . . . Without the hope of a transformation to come, the pain of answered prayer would be unbearable, it would mean the negation of faith . . . It is in this context that the meaning of "answered" prayers should be understood. They are not transactions complete in themselves, but signs of hope; signs which are the possession not only of the one whose prayer is answered, but of the whole community of faith, and so even of the one whose prayer remained unanswered.[21]

Epperly argues for a cosmology in which God, while active in the world, is not the sole cause of any event. He outlines a multiciplity of factors which influence health and well-being, in addition to "the divine will toward wholeness," and notes:

> The healing that is needed emerges from this lively and dynamic matrix of events. When prayer is not answered or healing does not occur in a strictly linear fashion, it is not due to God's arbitrary decision or lack of concern. Rather, it is due to the interplay of a constellation of events, in which one or more of the many factors may be the source of the failure.[22]

He sees prayer as having a global impact, shaping the environment of health both for the world and for the one being prayed for.

He notes Dossey's assertion (in *Healing Words*) that "thy will be done" prayers are more effective than specifically directed prayers, and suggests that "active openness to the divine will aligns us to what is best for the universe and the planet, part and whole, and contributes wholeheartedly to God's specific as well as general purposes in the universe."[23]

I greatly like Epperly's approach, but I cannot help but be struck by how unhelpful the majority of the patients with whom I work would find that perspective. After working here for 10 years, the pervasive negative effects of serious, persistent mental illness are concrete for me, no longer an abstraction. I have watched the deterioration of too many of the people I met when I first came here; others are hanging on, and others have been helped significantly by new medications and psychiatric rehabilitation programs. But even when help has come, the years of illness have taken their toll. Too often, energy which might otherwise have gone into growth has been consumed by survival.

It is difficult to talk of spiritual maturity without sounding judgmental, but maturity is an important dynamic in a life of prayer. Smith and Smith, in response to the film *Shadowlands,* the story of the marriage of C. S. Lewis and Joy Gresham, reflect on the limited nature of Joy's prayers, "a year or so of happiness with Jack at least." They note, "Prayers asking for something less than a cure are not uncommon among mature Christians."[24]

Louis Gruber equates genuine spirituality with radical surrender, including surrender to the will of God, and notes:

> . . . false spirituality is almost always the disguised attempt to control someone or something . . . False spirituality in the church, often showing these very characteristics, is the attempt to control God, oneself, situations, or other people through the use of (apparently) Christian prayer, terminology and practices. It is a "spirituality" of the ego, rather than of the Holy Spirit.[25]

Michael McCullough[26] offers a parallel understanding, suggesting that maturity in faith may lead people to value intimacy with God more than answers to specific prayers.

This perspective is hard to attain when all of one's energies must go into simply surviving, and it is particularly hard to attain when one's experiences in life make it difficult to form attachments with others, much less with God. Patients continue to make requests for specific prayers; I include these in my prayers for them, but more often I simply try to lift them up to God, seeing them surrounded by the light of Christ's love. I don't pray for all the patients; there are 180 of them and the time required would be considerable. But more importantly, I feel it would be intrusive to many of them, those who have told us that religion is not part of their lives. The tradition in the church is that one prays for those who request prayers in one way or another, or for those to whom one is sufficiently connected to request prayer on their behalf. I operate on the assumption that people who understand themselves to be Christian want the prayers of other Christians; I generally would ask before praying for someone of another faith, or no faith.

The question of "intrusiveness" has not been considered in any of the research thus far; I hope it will be in the future. I also hope that future research might take seriously Epperly's multiplicity of factors which shape health, though I realize it would be a significant challenge to integrate them into a study. McCullough[27] raises the question of how religious commitment on the part of those prayed for might affect treatment efficacy, and this could include the question of whether the efficacy of intercessory prayer is influenced by religious commitment.

In spite of my questions about Dossey' paper, I am grateful for it and for the opportunity to reflect upon it. I hope that this volume may help to instigate discussion within the community of faith and between faith and medicine.

AUTHOR NOTE

After I submitted this response, I read *Forgotten Truths: The Common Vision of the World's Religions* (1992; Harper). I wish I had read it earlier for it offers a way of synthesizing and ordering the domains of religion and science. For those interested in this topic, I strongly recommend it.

In writing this article, I have realized again the importance of the faith community in whose midst I work. I have greatly appreciated the thoughts and comments of numerous members of this community and most especially the assistance of chaplain intern Cathy Johnanson in locating and collecting references.

REFERENCES

1. Nahama Leibowitz. *Studies in Shemot (Exodus) Part I*; translated and adapted from the Hebrew by Aryeh Newman. (Jerusalem: The World Zionist Organization, 1981), 285.

2. Nahama Leibowitz, 286.

3. Nahama Leibowitz, 286.

4. Keith Stewart Thomson. "The revival of experiments on prayer." *American Scientist* 1996; 84:532-534.

5. Gerhard Kittel and Gerhard Friedrich. *Theological Dictionary of the New Testament*. Translated by Geoffrey W. Bromley. (Stuttgart, Germany: Wm. B. Eerdmans Publishing Co., 1968), Vol. VI, 32.

6. Lawrence LeShan. *The Medium, the Mystic and the Physicist* (New York: Viking Press, 1974).

7. David J. Hufford. "Epistemologies in religious healing." *The Journal of Medicine and Philosophy* 1993; 18:175-194.

8. David J. Hufford, 178.

9. David J. Hufford, 178.

10. Jeremy T. Law. "Questions People Ask: 3. Prayer: Problem or possibility?" *The Expository Times* 1995; 107(1):4-10, 10.

11. Leonard I. Sweet. *Health and Medicine in the Evangelical Tradition.* (Valley Forge, PA.: Trinity Press International, 1994).

12. Thomas Furman Hewitt. "The redefinition of intercessory prayer in contemporary theology." *Perspectives in Religious Studies* 1975; 2:65-80.

13. Bruce G. Epperly. "To pray or not to pray: Reflections on the intersection of prayer and medicine." *Journal of Religion and Health* 1995; 34(2):141-148.

14. Samuel Calian Carnegie. "Prayer during seminary years and beyond." *Perspectives* 1995; 16-18.

15. Daniel Day Lewis. *The Minister and The Care of Souls* (New York: Harper & Row, 1961), 116.

16. Bruce G. Epperly, 144.

17. Larry Dossey. *Healing Words* (San Francisco: HarperSanFrancisco, 1993), xvii.

18. Bernard N. Nathanson. Book review of *Healing Words: The Power of Prayer and the Practice of Medicine. First Things* 1994; 43:57-59, 57.

19. William E. Lesher. "Intercessory prayer: A spirituality for modern times." *Currents in Theology and Mission* 1993; 20:80a-80b.

20. Frank Hijikata. Book review of *Healing Words: The Power of Prayer and the Practice of Medicine. The Journal of Religion and Psychical Research* 1996; 19:112-115.

21. Jeremy T. Law, 10.

22. Bruce G. Epperly, 144.

23. Bruce G. Epperly, 147.

24. A. C. Smith and L. K. R. Smith. " 'Shadowlands,' Reflections on prayers for people who are seriously ill." *The Expository Times* 1995; 106:265-267, 266.

25. Louis N. Gruber. "True and false spirituality: A framework for christian behavioral medicine." *Journal of Psychology and Christianity* 1995; 14(2):133-140.

26. Michael E. McCullough. "Prayer and health: Conceptual issues, research review and research agenda." *Journal of Psychology and Theology* 1995; 23(1):15-29.

27. Michael E. McCullough.

A Response to Larry Dossey:
The Prayers of the Faithful:
Prayer as a Metaphor
for Medicine and Healing

William R. DeLong, MDiv

I learned to pray to a God that heard my prayers and would act upon them "according to his will." As I matured through the blessings and disappointments of life, I began to see prayer as a kind of piñata. At times I swung the bat of prayer and hit the swinging animal that held my hopes and dreams and at other times I would swing the bat wondering if the piñata God was there.

What I learned about prayer and faith is changing because of science. The cooperation of science and theology is at an all time high. Scholars in both areas are turning their attention to consider the effects of the scientific method and its implications for faith.[1] Larry Dossey's work is an example of the mutual interests of science and theology. Yet tension surfaces when we consider the more traditional and foundational areas of each. Prayer is just such an example. Dossey does a fine job in this paper describing the long-

William R. DeLong is Director of Chaplaincy Services and Pastoral Education, BroMenn Healthcare, Bloomington, IL 61702.

[Haworth co-indexing entry note]: "A Response to Larry Dossey: The Prayers of the Faithful: Prayer as a Metaphor for Medicine and Healing." DeLong, William R. Co-published simultaneously in *Journal of Health Care Chaplaincy* (The Haworth Pastoral Press, an imprint of The Haworth Press, Inc.) Vol. 7, No. 1/2, 1998, pp. 63-71; and: *Scientific and Pastoral Perspectives on Intercessory Prayer: An Exchange Between Larry Dossey, M.D. and Health Care Chaplains* (ed: Larry VandeCreek) The Haworth Pastoral Press, an imprint of The Haworth Press, Inc., 1998, pp. 63-71; and: *Scientific and Pastoral Perspectives on Intercessory Prayer: An Exchange Between Larry Dossey, M.D. and Health Care Chaplains* (ed: Larry VandeCreek) Harrington Park Press, an imprint of The Haworth Press, Inc., 1998, pp. 63-71. Single or multiple copies of this article are available for a fee from The Haworth Document Delivery Service [1-800-342-9678, 9:00 a.m. - 5:00 p.m. (EST). E-mail address: getinfo@haworth.com].

63

standing impasse between theology and science when each considers prayer.

As with most topics in a post-modern age, my view of prayer seems to change depending upon my vantage point. At times I understand prayer to be the process by which I move toward the Holy Other in an attempt to make my "petitions" known to God. I understand this perspective as my gut level need to connect to something "more than"–a transcendent reality greater than my own thoughts and intrapsychic process. At other times, such as when I pray with a family in the intensive care unit, I reflect on prayer as a resource of comfort, a familiar ritual that brings healing in a variety of ways in moments when profound healing is needed. Yet at other times, such as when I read Larry Dossey's paper, I am confronted with the "observed effects" of prayer.

I want to consider in this paper how the vantage point of an observer (attitudes, assumptions, bias, etc.) effects how we understand prayer.[2] *In particular, I want to reflect upon how the act and intention of observing the effects of prayer changes that which is observed.* How does our desire to demonstrate whether prayer has any "effect whatsoever" change the nature of prayer itself? Finally, and perhaps most importantly, I want to consider how the conclusions made from observing the effects of prayer alter the focus of the dialogue between spirituality and medicine. In so doing, I will be taking an epistemological look at Dr. Dossey's challenging paper. I hope to respond to Dossey's concluding challenges to join in a "genuine dialogue between medicine and spirituality," and to "take these scientific results seriously and craft your own response to them."

Any interpretive task is met with preconditions that change the very nature of the observed object. We learn from hermeneutics that everyone brings something to the task of interpretation, "A person who is trying to understand a text is always performing an act of projecting. He projects before himself a meaning for the text. Again, the latter emerges only because he is reading the text with particular expectations in regard to a certain meaning."[3] Our desire to find comfort in the reality of prayer through the use of scientific methods will change how we understand prayer. The question is how will it change? I believe Dossey suggests three possible implications.

First, prayer will become organized around a kind of "cause and effect" relationship, weakening the primacy of relating to God through prayer. Second, prayer will become a tool for the use of the, albeit fervent, prayer practitioner, lending itself more to a technique than a process. Finally our definition of prayer will become so broad that it will lose much of the meaning it has for many people. *As we move toward a more broad and expansive definition of prayer, we will also lose some of the qualities that make it an important part of the pastoral care in many religious traditions. In each of these ways prayer becomes more distorted and vague, and less valuable or efficacious.*

Prayer is an integral part of the human religious experience. Prayer in the Judeo-Christian tradition divides into various "types" of prayer based on the "intended" purpose of the prayer. Karl Rahner describes different aspects of prayer historically recognized in the Christian faith, "adoration, praise, thanksgiving, penitence, oblation, intercession, and petition."[4] In a recent article on prayer, Daniel Grossoehme describes these seven different types of prayer and their use in the hospital setting.[5] By examining prayers written in a hospital chapel prayer book, Grossoehme determined that "the vast majority of the prayers (fifty-one of seventy-five) were intercessory."[6] Intercessory prayer as defined by Dossey is ". . . communication with the Absolute" and I agree. It is this very point that unites the various forms of prayer identified in the Christian tradition. Prayers change depending upon the purpose for praying, such as when asking for forgiveness (penitence) or giving thanks for prayers already answered (thanksgiving). Yet the basic structure of prayer remains the same. The subject in each of these prayer forms is "the Absolute." The other participant in the "communication," is God. With the shift of focus from the process and relationship to the measurable outcome, prayer falls more into the realm of *techne*, a technique used to reach a particular end. (It is no coincidence that this is the primary method used in medicine today.)

After defining the term of prayer rather broadly, Dossey broadens the definition again by introducing the term "distant intentionality." The definition becomes further enlarged with supposed synonyms to prayer such as "concentrated," and "mental effort." Although the ensuing discussion of parapsychology is interesting and in my opinion correct, it does tend to shift the focus away from what I believe is a necessary defining characteristic of prayer, namely the God/human participants in the dialogue. Because of the broad definition, I am not always sure Dossey is talking about prayer. Prayer as I understand and practice it requires that I have some intentionality in communicating with God. Two core principles lay at the heart of prayer; human freedom (intentionality) and human relating to the Divine (transcendence). Not all prayer-like communication is prayer. For example, I may sit on my floor at home and meditate or focus on a particular desire of mine, say the health and well-being of my children. Yet, I would not consider this an act of intercessory prayer. Even if the result of my meditation in fact provided health and well-being for my children, it was not, in my opinion, a communication with the Absolute.

In this case observing the effect of prayer shifts the focus from the process of prayer as communication with the Divine Other. In so doing Dossey sufficiently obscures one of the defining characteristics of the process of prayer, "communication with the Absolute." Central to my understanding of prayer and diminished in Dossey's paper is prayer as an act of relationality. Regardless of the effect (a difficult thing to do for those in the medical sciences) the process is centrally and I believe, definitively, a process of relating with God.

Several Biblical references help us gain understanding of prayer as a relational experience. Consider Abraham's negotiations with Yahweh in Gen 18:23-33; and Jesus' pleading dialogue with the Father in Gesthsemane and again when we encounter the disciples asking Jesus to "teach us to pray" (Luke 11:1). Karl Rahner describes several necessary aspects of prayer.[7] Rahner sees prayer as a response to God's call and a free act by the human other,

> All prayer is wholly the gift of God . . . Man [sic] is not a machine kept in motion by God. He is free, and there can be no question of prayer unless it is rooted in man's freedom, an action in which he is personally responsible. These two aspects, which both take in the total act of human prayer must be clearly distinguished.[8]

In each of these instances it is the relationship that defines the act of prayer. Prayer links the human relating to God, and the freedom of human choice or intentionality in that relating.

By concentrating upon the effect of prayer Dossey proposes a very different set of partners in the prayer relationship. Dossey's emphasis on effect or outcomes almost exclusively concentrates on the partnership of the person who prays and the measurable effect on the target of prayer. Because of this the relational interaction of prayer as "communication with the Absolute" is diminished and almost disregarded.

Another concern with Dossey's attention to the effects of prayer is a hermeneutic one. First, what is the lens by which we understand the need to quantify the effects of prayer in order to demonstrate the efficacy of it? Second, how do we begin to frame the broader discussion of spirituality in health care when we use scientific methods as the basis for that discussion? What happens to prayer when we act on our need to quantify the effects of prayer in order to have confidence in its use with patients and family members? Dossey hints at his preference for a quantifiable lens for justifying the use of prayer by saying "In this paper I intend to challenge chaplains to take prayer seriously, to take it seriously *because* of what science is discovering" (italics mine).

The scientific method has provided us with much. At various times it is the friend of pastoral care providers and at other times a misunderstood and hence distrusted method. Chaplains and other pastoral care providers benefit by their increased understanding and use of the behavioral sciences. Through quantifying the needs of patients, hospital chaplaincy staffs have increased. Quantitative studies have demonstrated where chaplains should focus their time in the hospitals. Double blind studies increase the understanding of chaplains and the effective use of their ministry.[9] In these ways the scientific method has been a friend. Yet, many of us live in the tension of blessing and curse with this method. I believe the curse of science has something to do with the degree that we rely on science to tell us what is true. Scientific methodology has acquired the role in our culture to separate truth from fiction. It has become the predominant lens by which we determine the veracity of our subjective experience. This is more pervasive in health care than in any other aspect of science. If it is not statistically relevant, then it is not real.

In the larger scientific arena, Thomas Kuhn points out the need for the observed data to support existing theory.[10] It is not uncommon for the theory to enable researchers to ignore data because it does not fit the theory. Our need to support the existing viewpoint is a part of the lens by which we consider new information. This is true in the medical sciences as well.

The effect this has on the practice of medicine was made clear in Norman Cousin's book *The Healing Heart*.[11] In his description of his own illness, Cousins pointed out the many times his symptoms were ignored because they did not fit the clinical picture of his disease. The predominant lens for determining reality in medicine has been the compatibility of the object with the known (read scientifically supported) theory. Yet, medicine received increasing critique for its inability to accept the patient's point of view. In light of this many physicians are now advocating listening to the patient's subjective reality of their symptoms as a primary part of the diagnostic process.[12] All of this has led to increased attention to the metaphors and the hermeneutic used in health care.

The need for a new hermeneutic in health care is increasingly clear. In many ways Dossey's own work vividly depicts this need.[13] Many are now casting about for metaphors that enlighten the healing task of medicine.[14] One of those concerned with this task from a hermeneutic perspective is Hans-George Gadamer in his fascinating new book *The Enigma of Health*. In this work Gadamer helps us understand how the method of science, when applied to other areas of human/God endeavors, changes how we understand the object of inquiry. His primary concern is to understand how the patient's understanding (hermeneutic) is disregarded in favor of the scientific assumption. Gadamer says:

> Now the experience which has been reworked by the sciences has, indeed, the merit of being verifiable and acquirable by everyone. But then, in addition, it raises the claim that on the basis of its methodological procedure it is the only certain experience, hence the only mode of knowing in which each and every experience is rendered truly legitimate. What we know from practical experience and the 'extra-scientific' do-

main must not only be subjected to scientific verification but also, should it hold its ground against this demand, belongs by this very fact to the domain of scientific research. There is in principle nothing which could not be subordinated in this manner to the competence of science.[15]

Gadamer points out that because of the power of the scientific method to explain and verify the object studied, the very nature of the studied object falls under the realm of the scientific. With Gadamer I question how the use of the scientific method to demonstrate the efficacy of prayer subordinates prayer itself to the scientific. When this happens, how does prayer change?

This leads me to my final concern with Dr. Dossey's position. Dossey seems to suggest in his paper that the larger dialogue of spirituality and health care should be predicated upon the foundations of the scientific method. By continuing the validation of reality through the scientific method, and extending that method to prayer itself, I believe Dossey encourages a process that will hinder the creation of new metaphors for health care, limit the possibility of a fresh paradigm for medicine and, in short, perpetuate what we already have.

In a helpful book on spiritual guidance, Carolyn Gratton imagines the wise spiritual guide to be one who "co-listens" with the client.[16] Co-listening may be one way to begin to think about the spiritual/medical dialogue. What would happen to our current model of medicine if we really began to practice the spiritual art of co-listening? What are patients and family members trying to say about the human condition and our need to feel God's presence in our life by questioning the way the scientific method has fashioned the medical model?

Co-listening in health care would mean that we listen to how the spiritual infuses the healing process. If we apply Gratton's words about the individual seeker of truth to the discussion of spirituality and medicine, and we consider ourselves as guides of this process, we can hear the implications of co-listening, "As co-listeners, guides can be alert for possible onesidedness, for spiritual opportunities that might otherwise be overlooked, and for the attunement or disharmony they sense in the person's resistance coming from the various polarities of the life field."[17] This notion itself leads us to think about a shared reality rather than splitting off the quantifiable from the numinous in human experience. Co-listening in health care would invite the physician to hear the subjective meanings of a person's illness. As Gadamer quotes in his book, the important question that is rarely asked in health care is "what does illness tell the one who is ill? Not so much, what does it tell the doctor, but rather, what does it tell the patient?"[18] Co-listening as a metaphor for the spiritual/medical dialogue allows for a process that would search for the root metaphors that could sustain an integrated approach to healing.

After all, religion, magic, and medicine shared the same early roots of medicine men and priests. If we continue to base this important dialogue on the results of empirical studies, then we really do not shift the foundation of the medical model. Andrew Weil says it well, "Science and intellect can show us mechanisms and details of physical reality–and that knowledge is surely of value–but they cannot unveil the deep mysteries."[19] Genuine dialogue will involve co-listening at the deepest levels of human experience. Co-listening as a prayerful experience for medicine, will become a process by which we seek to find that which is truly new, a transformation in our understanding about how we learn and act about healing and health. Co-listening will allow us to predicate a new model for healing on both the quantifiable and the subjective, relying upon both to describe the reality of health and healing. Like the disciples of old, I too must learn . . . "Lord, teach us to pray."

REFERENCES

1. Thomas F. Torrance. *Transformation and Convergence in the Frame of Knowledge* (Grand Rapids: Eerdmans, 1984); Michael Polany. *Knowing and Being* (Chicago: University of Chicago Press, 1969); James Loder and W. Jim Neidhardt. *The Knight's Move* (Colorado Springs: Helmers and Howard, 1992).

2. This is our pre-understanding that we bring to any interpretive task. Hans-George Gadamer called this "fore-meaning." Hans-George Gadamer. *Truth and Method* (New York: Crossroads, 1985), 237.

3. Hans-George Gadamer, 236.

4. Karl Rahner. *Dictionary of Theology* (New York: Crossroads, 1985), 404.

5. Daniel H. Grossoehme. "Prayer reveals belief: images of God from hospital prayer." *Journal of Pastoral Care* 1996; 50(1);33-39.

6. Daniel H. Grossoehme, 34.

7. Karl Rahner, 1275.

8. Karl Rahner, 1278.

9. Larry VandeCreek. *Spiritual Needs and Pastoral Services: Readings in Research.* (Journal of Pastoral Care Publications, Inc, 1995). This is an excellent resource that demonstrates how scientific research has been influential in pastoral care and counseling.

10. Thomas Kuhn. *The Structure of Scientific Revolutions.* (Chicago: University of Chicago Press, 1966).

11. Norman Cousins. *The Healing Heart.* (New York: Norton Books), 1979.

12. Consider the works of Bernie Siegel. *Love, Medicine and Miracles* (New York: HarperCollins), 1988; M. Scott Peck. *The Road Less Traveled* (Cutchogue: Buccaneer Books, 1978) and others.

13. Larry Dossey. *Meaning and Medicine* (New York: Bantam Books, 1991). I was surprised that Dossey did not reference this work more in this paper. In particular see his section on meaning and health.

14. See Andrew Weil. *Health and Healing* (Boston: Houghton Mifflin, 1995).

15. Hans-George Gadamer. *The Enigma of Health* (Stanford: The Stanford University Press, 1996), 2.

16. Carolyn Gratton. *The Art of Spiritual Guidance* (New York: Crossroad, 1993).

17. Carolyn Gratton, 52.

18. Hans-Goerge Gademer, 76.

19. Andrew Weil, 46.

A Chaplain's Response
to Prayer, Medicine, and Science:
The New Dialogue

Carol Anne Schroder, MDiv

My personal experiences with the healing benefits of prayer led me to hospital ministry. The most dramatic test of my response to healing prayer occurred in my Junior year as a student at San Francisco Theological Seminary. I agree with Dr. Dossey's premise about testing prayer in one's own life, "People test prayer in their individual lives, and one's life is the most important laboratory of all." Nine years ago, on April 7, 1988, my gynecologist diagnosed me with ovarian cancer. He told me I needed urgent life-saving surgery due to a fast-growing tumor. One week before my surgery, I prepared to die. I shared the bad news of my cancer diagnosis with my friends, family, students, and professors. I prepared a will and wrote goodbye letters to my three daughters. My outlook was grim.

I gave each of my children a heart locket and a small picture of me to remind them of my love. At this time I was separated from their father. Three seminaries, six churches, family members, and

---

Carol Anne Schroder is affiliated with Clinical Pastoral Services, University of California–Davis Medical Center, Sacramento, CA 95670.

[Haworth co-indexing entry note]: "A Chaplain's Response to Prayer, Medicine, and Science: The New Dialogue." Schroder, Carol Anne. Co-published simultaneously in *Journal of Health Care Chaplaincy* (The Haworth Pastoral Press, an imprint of The Haworth Press, Inc.) Vol. 7, No. 1/2, 1998, pp. 73-86; and: *Scientific and Pastoral Perspectives on Intercessory Prayer: An Exchange Between Larry Dossey, M.D. and Health Care Chaplains* (ed: Larry VandeCreek) The Haworth Pastoral Press, an imprint of The Haworth Press, Inc., 1998, pp. 73-86; and: *Scientific and Pastoral Perspectives on Intercessory Prayer: An Exchange Between Larry Dossey, M.D. and Health Care Chaplains* (ed: Larry VandeCreek) Harrington Park Press, an imprint of The Haworth Press, Inc., 1998, pp. 73-86. Single or multiple copies of this article are available for a fee from The Haworth Document Delivery Service [1-800-342-9678, 9:00 a.m. - 5:00 p.m. (EST). E-mail address: getinfo@haworth.com].

friends prayed for my successful surgery. I was touched by these compassionate prayers, which blessed me with a rapid recovery. One month later I returned to watch seniors graduate. I have experienced hospital ministry from both sides of the hospital bed. Since then prayer has speeded my recovery from additional health challenges.

Years later I shared my healing lesson with my mother and father. In June, 1991, my father, a retired ophthalmologist, survived surgical removal of a cancerous kidney. When his doctor prescribed a two-month course of radiation treatments, he expressed fear of the unpleasant side effects of radiation. Throughout his radiation therapy my mother and I prayed and visualized God's healing light and angels surrounding him. Amazingly, my father, a skeptical scientist, did not suffer any side effects. In fact, he continued to swim at the YMCA three times a week.

PERSONAL ENCOUNTERS
WITH THE HEALING BENEFITS OF PRAYER

In Dr. Dossey's commentary he challenges chaplains to take their prayers with patients seriously.

> I know that chaplains pray with patients and their families. I do not know how seriously they take that ministry. Some, perhaps many, may regard it as an obligation or a purely religious performance in response to expectations. In this paper I intend to challenge chaplains to take prayer seriously, to take it seriously because of what science is discovering.

I do take my prayer with hospital patients seriously! I have never used a canned healing prayer. However, before I begin my prayer work with a patient I assess his or her spiritual need and background. Every prayer is tailored to the individual patient, according to his or her spiritual belief. My pastoral role is to support the patient's own spirituality. I am their spiritual companion and fellow pray-er.

Often at patients' requests I provide them with the holy book of their choice. Our pastoral care office is stocked with multi-lingual

Catholic and Protestant Bibles, Books of Mormon, Korans, as well as Buddhist literature. I learn about my patients' faith beliefs by asking questions and carefully listening to their spiritual points of view. Spiritual assessment is a common practice among all chaplains.

I regard each patient as my spiritual teacher. It makes no difference to me whether a patient calls God: Jehovah, Yahweh, Allah, Buddha, or Jesus. I've learned to have a broader view of God, whom I believe has many names. In my pastoral care I choose to focus on the individual patient's relationship with his/her divinity. Slowly, over time, I develop a pastoral relationship with each patient. Normally, I'm not in the habit of giving "quick-stop" healing prayers.

One significant example of prayer-at-work is the case of a ten-year-old girl in the Pediatric Unit who suffered from a rare form of brain cancer. When I met her, she was recovering from surgical removal of her cancerous tumor. She was unable to talk or walk. I prayed with the girl and her parents for her healing. I gave her a small angel prayer card, which she kept under her pillow. The Catholic chaplain and I collaborated in a concentrated prayer routine, with profound results in a very short time. She responded rapidly, and soon was able to talk and play with other children. I followed the child over a year and a half while she underwent radiation and chemotherapy treatment. She is now in remission. Another example from the dozens during my tenure at this hospital, was the forty-year-old single woman, terrified the night before brain aneurysm surgery, who called for me in the middle of the night. I rushed to her bedside and prayed with her for hours in the Neuro Intensive Care Unit. She survived the surgery, and I visited her daily until her release. This Protestant patient returned to church and began to renew her relationship with a community of believers. A year later, she asked for prayer again to help her face a second aneurysm surgery, which two doctors advised would take them at least six hours. They warned her that she could be blinded, paralyzed, or even die in the process. Before this second surgery her friends and I placed our hands on her and prayed that the Lord would spare her life if it was His will. The surgery was a smashing success, and she was back in her room within three hours! She left the hospital three days later.

Still another miraculous recovery was the case of a nine-year-old boy who had been hit by a train, and was not expected to live. I met him in the Pediatric Special Care Unit shortly after his life-or-death orthopedic and brain surgeries. His mother and I sat near the unconscious boy's bed. She asked me to pray to Allah with her for his recovery, which I did. In follow-up visits I brought her a Koran to help her meditate according to her Muslim faith. A few days after my initial visit I returned to find the boy had been transferred to the Rehab floor. He was conscious and talking, and insisted on reading a book I'd brought for him. Within two weeks he discarded his casts and exceeded expectations in speech and physical therapy. He soon returned to school. His mother and he are convinced that Allah healed him. These examples illustrate the benefits of healing prayer in conjunction with medical treatment, for a natural, if not overnight, successful outcome. In a hospital environment the chaplain works as a member of a team, consisting of nurses, physicians, social workers, physical/speech therapists, and psychologists. Each member of the team contributes to the final healing process. Frequently, in a life/death situation, medical staff will request pastoral counseling for themselves. I have been privileged to conduct a memorial service for one medical staff team-member who died unexpectedly. The spirit of this team relationship is one of mutual respect and cooperation.

PRAYER IS A CONVERSATION WITH GOD

As a chaplain I have encountered patients from such diverse cultures as Vietnam, South America, Mexico, Africa and the Middle East, as well as U.S., Asian, Native American, Black, and other minorities. This medical center is a melting pot of cultures, religions, and socio-economic groups. The patients' spiritual perspectives are as multi-faceted as the cultures themselves.

I have learned to take an open-minded view toward patients' spiritual practices. *I have never encountered a patient who believed that God was a remote parent figure!* Dr. Dossey's misperception of a rigid limited view of God in American culture does not match my experience. In the present lead paper in this volume, he writes, "Prayer is talking aloud or to yourself to a white, male, cosmic parent figure who prefers to be addressed in English."

When I pray with patients for their healing, I have observed that as patients reach out to God they begin to feel comforted and reassured by a loving presence. Their illness forces them to rediscover or renew their relationship with God, and in the dark night of their soul they wrestle with the cosmic meaning of life. Kenneth Woodward, in *Newsweek Magazine*, comments on the motivation of pray-ers,

> According to recent studies at NORC, a research center, by Andrew M. Greeley, the sociologist-novelist-priest, more than three quarters (78 percent) of all Americans pray at least once a week; more than half (57%) report praying at least once a day. Indeed, Greeley finds that even among the 13 percent of Americans who are atheists or agnostics, nearly one in five still prays daily, siding, it seems with Pascal, and wagering that there is a God who hears them.
>
> Some of these prayers are born *in extremis*; there are few atheists in cancer wards or on unemployment lines. But in allegedly rootless, materialistic, self-centered America, there is also a hunger for a personal experience of God that prayer seeks to satisfy.[1]

Wherever I walk on my hospital rounds I meet people from all walks of life who pray to God for help with work or health challenges. A nurse, physician, or social worker who contacts a chaplain to visit a fearful or anxious patient, is expressing belief in the possibility that a chaplain's prayer will help allay a patient's upcoming surgery or possible death.

In another *Newsweek* article (March 31, 1997), Kenneth Woodward again reaffirms that most American adults pray.

> It is remarkable that in millenial America, where public cynicism seemingly knows no bounds and the coin of the mass-culture is cheap, ironic detachment, trust in God persists. The prayers keep coming–for health, safety, love and, to a remarkable degree, for others.[2]

Dr. Dossey's sterile definition of God left me cold and serves to widen the gap between medicine and religion. My own version of God is that of a warm, compassionate, and unconditionally loving presence who can be reached day or night, alone or in community with others. My God is very accessible. On the other hand, Dr. Dossey places God at a distance, "Prayer is communication with the Absolute."

Most pray-ers talk to God silently in their mind, or aloud with like-minded believers. I felt relieved to read Dossey's redefinition of prayer in his book, *Prayer Is Good Medicine*:

> In it's simplest form, *prayer is an attitude of the heart*—a matter of *being,* not doing. Prayer is the desire to contact the Absolute, however, it may be confused when we experience the need to enact this connection. We are praying, whether or not we use words.[3]

My human condition unites me with all my sisters and brothers who lie on a bed of pain. Henri Nouwen, in his book, *The Wounded Healer,* reminds me to transform my woundedness into a healing relationship in my ministry.

> On the one hand, no minister can keep his own experience of life from those he wants to help. Nor should he want to keep it hidden . . . making one's own wounds a source of healing, therefore, does not call for a sharing as superficial personal pain but for constant willingness to see one's own pain and suffering as rising from the depth of the human condition, which all men share.[4]

Howard Rice, a retired chaplain of the San Francisco Theological Seminary, in his book *Reformed Spirituality, An Introduction For Believers,* discusses the theological perspective of prayer. I agree, because prayer has been a natural response to my human condition. Rice aptly describes how humans reach out to God for comfort when they are in trouble.

> It is natural for us all to pray to God for those things we need most. We try to get God to see things our way and to answer

our requests favorably. We cannot and should not avoid such kinds of prayer. When we are in trouble we naturally cry out to God for safety, health, or relief from danger. There are many examples in Scripture as an effort to get God to do something which a person or group needs. Prayers for rain, prayers for success of armies in battle, prayers for the end of pestilence, and prayers for long life and good health are common to all people.[5]

Supernatural Aspects of Prayer

I agree with Dossey's assertion that parapsychology and religion are interactive. No stronger proof exists than seemingly inexplicable Near Death Experiences (NDE). Thousands of NDE's have been documented in books by such well-known authors as Raymond Moody, M.D., Melvin Morse, M.D., Betty Eadie, Dannion Brinkley, Betty Malz, and Maurice Rawlings, M.D. In the present paper, Dossey discusses the mystical consequences of praying:

> In parapsychology experience, individuals often actually pray or enter a sacred, reverential, prayer-like state of mind to accomplish their task. On the other hand, when people pray, they often have paranormal experiences, such as telepathy, clairvoyance, or precognition.

In addition, I support Dossey's research undertaken by the British clergy, in which psychical phenomena seem to be meaningful to Christians in life and death. I recommend reading the following books written by people who have experienced supernatural glimpses of Heaven or the spirits of deceased loved ones:

- Raymond A. Moody, M.D. *Life After Life and Reflections On Life After Life* (New York: Guideposts, 1975).
- Melvin Morse, M.D., *Closer To The Light* (New York: Villard Books, 1990).
- Betty J. Eadie. *Embraced By The Light* (California: Gold Leaf Press, 1992).
- Dannion Brinkley. *Saved By The Light* (New York: Harper Collins, 1994).

- Betty Malz. *My Glimpse Of Eternity* (New Jersey: Chosen Books, 1977).
- Maurice F. Rawlings. *To Hell And Back* (Tennessee: Thomas Nelson, 1993).

Betty Eadie, Dannion Brinkley, and Betty Malz describe their mystical NDE out-of-body adventures after they were pronounced dead. The memory of their supernatural trips into a spiritual realm continues to reinforce the spiritual belief that they are souls who are having a human experience. They believe that they will die only after they have completed their mission on earth. They have no fear of death.

Physicians Raymond Moody, Melvin Morse, and Maurice Rawlings have recorded countless interviews with NDE patients. I also have personally talked with seriously ill or dying patients who claim to have seen deceased loved ones or angels. These visions invariably bring comfort and reassurance to the people. Children freely describe the angelic visitors whom they insist have come to their room. They do not regard such experiences as odd or unusual. Adults, however, reluctantly disclose their unearthly visitations, only after they feel able to trust that I'll take them seriously.

POSITIVE TEST RESULTS OF PRAYER

Prayer and parapsychology join together when healers, motivated by their compassionate healing love for people and animals, witness the powerful transformative effects of their prayers. I concur with Dr. Dossey's claim in his paper that love has been uncovered in laboratory experiments of prayer.

> Subjects in parapsychology often experience feelings that are central to prayer, such as love, empathy, compassion, and a central connectedness, oneness and unity with the object to influence . . . In them love seems to function as a form of intercession–literally, a go-between–that unites the object and the object being influenced. If love is crucial to the success of psi experiments, and if "God Is Love," then the Almighty appears to be less nervous than some believers entering the parapsychology lab.

In my work as a chaplain I have encountered positive attitudes among the medical staff about the benefits of prayer. So far, in my personal hospital "lab," I have never met anyone who believed it was blasphemous to test God. I have seen patients and family members receive a sense of hope when they turn to God in prayer. In spite of the outcome, healing or non-healing of the patient's medical condition, they persist in turning to God for their care. I have worked with dying patients who, after healing prayer in which I placed him in God's compassionate arms, are able to stop struggling, let go, and peacefully, spiritually, travel to God's lighted home.

My bias and perhaps my limitation as a non-scientist is that I refuse to cling to a total faith only in medication or medical procedure for healing patients. Instead, I have an open mind about the possibility of spiritual healing, in spite of negativity on the part of medical staff. For example, a physician called me to pray with a patient whom he believed would die within the hour. The patient was in intensive care, bleeding internally, and asked me to pray with him and his wife for healing. After I prayed with them, I left, and returned the next day to discover that the patient had been transferred to a regular unit. I met him and his wife as they walked together in the hallway. What a delightful surprise!

I am a Christian pastoral caregiver who models my ministry after the healing ministry of Jesus Christ. Morton Kelsey, a noted theologian summarizes my perception of Jesus as a man, both divine and human, whose compassionate touch and words of authority delivered emotionally, physically, and spiritually ill from their crippling circumstances. I admire Jesus' ministry of presence.

> Jesus used many different actions to heal the sick who came to him. He called upon the faith of the person who needed help, he touched the sick person, he uttered commands, he used various physical media . . . His most common means of healing was by speaking words and touching the sick person with his hands.[6]

My guidebook for hospital ministry rests on the miraculous healing stories of the New Testament. I believe that the Holy Spirit working in Biblical times is still working today. Mysticism is alive and well–ask any chaplain. In a way, the healing skills of physicians miraculously heal patients who would have died in ancient times. Miracles, whether performed by doctors or ministers are still miracles; and miracles are mystical by definition.

Jesus modeled a healing persona. His compassion, acceptance, and understanding of desperate human needs, healed people when they *believed* they could be healed. Faith in God is an essential element. The New Testament is filled with healing stories about Jesus, his disciples, and followers.

> A leper came to him, begging him, and kneeling, he said to him, 'If you choose, you can make me clean.' Moved with pity, Jesus stretched out his hand and touched him, and said to him, 'I do choose. Be made clean.' Immediately the leprosy left him and he was made clean.[7]

CHARISMATIC HEALING PRAYER

After graduation from Seminary I became involved with Presbyterian, Catholic, and Baptist charismatic healing groups. These groups were open to members of their respective churches and the general public. The monthly services were structured so that any individual requesting healing prayers could be blessed or anointed by selected healing teams. After the worship leader gave a brief homily and led the audience in hymns and a prayer, he/she invited those who sought healing to step forward for a blessing. One member of the team anointed the subject with holy oil and placed a cross on his/her brow, as prescribed by the healing prayer of James 5:13-16. Then team members gently placed their hands upon the person and prayed aloud for his or her healing. While there is some controversy, especially among traditionalists, over this type of service I have been both recipient and participant of such healing teams and know that many enjoy a high rate of success.

Agnes Sanford, a renowned Christian healer and author of *The Healing Light* and *The Healing Touch Of God,* affirmed that would-be healers who have faith in God's power to heal will be successful in their prayer healing ministries. She encourages healers to follow a healing formula.

Thus one might say that the first step in the prayer faith is the choosing; the second step is the seeing–and the third step is the speaking . . . in every case where Our Lord healed, He spoke the word that actually calls into being, or draws toward one an essence of power: a living, moving energy that God sends forth to accomplish His will. This energy is as actual as the energy of electricity or of cosmic rays or X-Rays or radiance. It can often be felt as the disciples of Emmaus felt it (Luke 24:32) as a tingling or as a heat, or as a certain movement in the air described as a rushing, mighty wind (Act 2:2).[8]

Francis MacNutt, a lay Catholic healer and former priest, conducts healing services in the U.S. and around the world. He explained about the powerful supernatural healing by the Holy Spirit in his books, *Overcome By The Spirit and Healing.*[9] He encourages members of his healing services to practice their healing skills on each other. He leads the audience in a mass healing prayer and asks each participant to place his or her hands on another person. He urges people to have faith in God, who will bless them with a gift of healing.

Charles and Myrtle Fillmore, who founded the Unity School of Christianity, practiced healing affirmation to help heal themselves of tuberculosis. Myrtle credited her healing gifts to the power of God within. She and her husband founded Silent Unity in Lee's Summit, Missouri. This is a 24-hour prayer group, composed of seventy people, who pray for anyone anywhere in the world, with merely a telephoned request. It is a non-denominational prayer ministry. This courageous 19th century couple developed a prayer technique, which they successfully practiced on themselves and others. Myrtle freely admitted the goal of Unity, "Unity is a school of religious investigation and experimentation."[10]

SPIRITUAL BREAKTHROUGHS IN MEDICINE

I agree with Dossey's assertion that lay people, scientists, and clergy are searching for concrete proof of the healing effect of prayer. If prayer could be bottled and dispensed like a prescription, the medical/religion debate would be resolved in a hurry. In his paper, Dossey examines the psychological roadblock which prevents medicine and religion from being a true partnership.

> Although we need more experimental data (scientists in every field say this), the major obstacle in taking intercessory prayer seriously is not, I think, a lack of empirical evidence. Our major difficulty is that we seem to be suffering from a failure of the imagination. Unable to see how prayer *could* work, too many people insist it can *not* work. Unless we learn to see the world in new ways, we shall remain unable to engage the evidence for intercessory prayer that already exists, and we shall be tempted to dismiss future evidence, no matter how strong it proves to be.

Andrew Weil, M.D., author of the best seller *Spontaneous Healing*, claims that there is a revolution brewing in modern medicine.[11] The advent of holistic medicine is providing alternatives such as prayer, meditation, acupuncture, herbal therapy and massage. A physician, Dr. Sam Benjamin, spiritualizes medicine at the Arizona Center for Health & Medicine.

> In (room) 16 (Grape seed) Sam Benjamin taps the last of 28 acupuncture needles into a man suffering from dizziness and back pain. Then he kneels near the man's head and begins to pray . . . Prayer is one of Benjamin's favorite tools. Sometimes he writes healing words from the Bible and tapes them to a patient's pillow before surgery. Does it work? He says, 'I think it does.'[12]

More and more physicians are taking a new, spiritual approach to medicine. It would take another paper to cover the growing number of resources written by physicians. The following list of books is a representative sample.

- Herbert Benson, M.D. *Timeless Healing, The Power And Biology Of Belief* (New York: Fireside Books, 1996).
- Deepak Chopra, M.D. *Creating Health* (New York: Houghton Mifflin, 1991).
- Deepak Chopra, M.D. *Quantum Healing* (New York: Bantam Books, 1990).

- Dean Ornish, M.D. *Reversing Heart Disease* (New York: Ballantine Books, 1990).

A NEW ALLIANCE OF MEDICINE AND PRAYER

In summary, my personal experience as a chaplain has served as a proving ground for the medical and religious professions in their almost adversarial roles in the practice of healing. My personal life furnished a foundation for my hospital ministry. I have seen a profound change in attitude on both sides, but especially in the new respect now being shown for religion by medical staff everywhere. Prayer is being taken more seriously these days than many people think, Dr. Larry Dossey included.

Dr. Dossey has brilliantly covered The New Dialogue, as his title suggests, from the medical and scientific standpoints. I've discussed it from my personal viewpoint as a chaplain. I think Religion, Medicine, and Science are closer together than ever before in the matter of benefits of prayer in healing. I feel privileged to have been in a position to witness miraculous recoveries among patients, which doctors themselves are unable to explain, except by divine intervention.

I have accepted Dr. Dossey's challenge to chaplains to take their prayer work seriously. I certainly do, and have never met a chaplain who was even slightly negative as to the effectiveness of his or her prayers. For me, God is a listening, personal Lord of Love, and embraces people of all cultures, races, and religions. I definitely have a broader view of Larry Dossey's "Absolute."

REFERENCES

1. Kenneth L. Woodward. "Talking to God." *Newsweek*. Jan. 6, 1992; Vol. CXIX, No. 1: 39-44; 39.

2. Kenneth L. Woodward. "Is God listening?" *Newsweek*. March 31, 1997, Vol. CXXIX, No. 13:57-65; 58.

3. Larry Dossey. *Prayer Is Good Medicine* (California: Harper, 1996), 83.

4. Henri J.M Nouwen. *The Wounded Healer* (New York: Image Books, 1979), 88.

5. Howard L. Rice. *Reformed Spirituality* (Kentucky: Westminster/John Knox Press, 1991), 72.

6. Morton T. Kelsey. *Healing and Christianity* (New York: Harper and Row), 79.

7. Mark 1:40-43.

8. Agnes Sanford. *The Healing Touch Of God* (New York: Ballantine Books, 1958), 43.

9. Francis MacNutt. *Overcome by the Spirit* (New Jersey: Chosen Books, 1990), 158.

10. Neal Vahle. *Torch Bearer To Light The Way* (California: Open View Press, 1996), p. 149.

11. Andrew Weil. *Spontaneous Healing* (NY: Ballentine Books, 1995), 65.

12. George Howe Colt. "See me, feel me, touch me, heal me," *Life* Sept. 1996. 35-51; 42.

A Buddhist Response to Larry Dossey

Madeline Ko-i Bastis, BCC

THE BUDDHIST PRACTICE OF PRAYER

Like many Americans who have embraced Buddhism, I was interested in Buddhist philosophy and psychology;[1] I was impressed by the Buddha's lack of dogmatism. He did not demand faith in what he had discovered, but exhorted others to find the truth for themselves.[2] As a well-educated, successful middle-aged American, I was not interested in devotion, ritual or prayer. After all, a famous Zen saying is, "If you meet the Buddha on the road, kill him."[3] I wanted to find the meaning of life for myself and spent many years sitting on the cushion (meditation practice) and ignored various devotional practices. *During my first unit of Clinical Pastoral Education (CPE) my refrain was, "We don't have prayer!" and if, as Dossey found, prayer is narrowly defined by many Americans as ". . . talking aloud or to yourself, to a white, male, cosmic parent figure who prefers to be addressed in English," then Buddhists don't pray.*

If one accepts Dossey's definition of prayer as "communication with the Absolute" then, in fact, Buddhists do pray. It is the prayer-

---

Madeline Ko-i Bastis is Founder and Director of Peaceful Dwelling Project, Inc., East Hampton, NY 11937.

[Haworth co-indexing entry note]: "A Buddhist Response to Larry Dossey." Bastis, Madeline Ko-i. Co-published simultaneously in *Journal of Health Care Chaplaincy* (The Haworth Pastoral Press, an imprint of The Haworth Press, Inc.) Vol. 7, No. 1/2, 1998, pp. 87-96; and: *Scientific and Pastoral Perspectives on Intercessory Prayer: An Exchange Between Larry Dossey, M.D. and Health Care Chaplains* (ed: Larry VandeCreek) The Haworth Pastoral Press, an imprint of The Haworth Press, Inc., 1998, pp. 87-96; and: *Scientific and Pastoral Perspectives on Intercessory Prayer: An Exchange Between Larry Dossey, M.D. and Health Care Chaplains* (ed: Larry VandeCreek) Harrington Park Press, an imprint of The Haworth Press, Inc., 1998, pp. 87-96. Single or multiple copies of this article are available for a fee from The Haworth Document Delivery Service [1-800-342-9678, 9:00 a.m. - 5:00 p.m. (EST). E-mail address: getinfo@haworth.com].

ful state of mind that is important, not the method. Some people sing hymns, others chant sutras; some clap their hands, others spin in circles; some sit in silence, others read prayers aloud. It is the intention that's important—the wish to communicate (or from a Buddhist point of view to *merge* or become one) with the Absolute. Clearly singing a pop song in the shower is not the same as singing a hymn with a congregation.

The two major schools of Buddhism are Theravada[4] and Mahayana.[5] The Theravada tradition, which originated in Southeast Asia has a long tradition of intercessory prayer. There is a practice of *Metta* (loving-kindness)[6] where the mediator sends good wishes to another by repeating phrases:

> May you be safe from inner and outer harm.
> May you be happy and peaceful.
> May you be strong and healthy.
> May you take care of yourself with joy.

Transference of merit is also important in Theravada Buddhism. The large monastic community in Southeast Asia depends solely on donations for survival and there is often a waiting list for lay people to prepare and offer the main meal of the day for the monks. One receives merit by performing an act of generosity and the merit can be transferred to one who has died. In making an offering, the practitioner acknowledges the Absolute, shows respect and gratitude to the monks who have devoted their lives to the Buddha's teachings and asks for blessings—usually the resolution of karma,[7] a peaceful death and an auspicious rebirth. One is reminded of the gifts of the Magi in the Christian tradition.

The Mahayana school has many sects: Pure Land, Tendai, Shingon and Mchiren Shoshu, as well as Tibetan (with several distinct lineages) and Zen. Having no personal experience of Pure Land,[8] Tendai,[9] Shingoni[10] and Nichiren Shoshu,[11] I suggest the references be checked for more information. All four are devotional schools with Nichiren Shoshu enjoying a particular popularity in America with more than 140,000 active members.[12] The main practice is chanting from the Lotus Sutra and repeating the phrase "Nam Myoho Renge Kyo" (Devotion to the Lotus Blossom of the Fine Dharma) while fingering a male (rosary) of 108 beads. One can chant for a new car, money, love, health for oneself or others.[13]

Since the chant is a mantra, the practitioner can become one with the Absolute.

The Tibetan schools are rich in devotion, ritual and prayer. There is Guru yoga[14] where through prayer and meditation one merges with the guru (teacher) who is considered to be the embodiment of Buddhahood. A practitioner can align the self with the Absolute by visualizing Buddhist deities in the elaborate form of mandala.[15] By concentrating on the intricate details of a mandala (all from memory) the notion of self is erased and union with the deity is achieved. Bowing practice also serves to empty the self so that there is alignment with the absolute and it is not unusual for serious practitioners to perform 1000 full prostrations during the day.

The *Phowa*[16] and *Tonglen*[17] practices seem closest to the Christian idea of prayer. *The Phowa is a visualization done for one who is dying or is already dead. First the practitioner quiets the mind and then visualizes the dying person merging with the source of all goodness and love. In other words, the dying person not only touches or communicates with the absolute but becomes one with it. We might call it "going home."* In Tonglen (giving and receiving), the practitioner takes on the suffering of another by visualizing it as black smoke. One breathes in the black suffering, purifies it and releases white healing air. This is in marked contrast to some New Age techniques where one inhales white light and expels pain. In Buddhism an acceptance of the dark side is necessary before one can truly experience the light. "The Identity of Relative and Absolute" a key Zen Buddhist sutra tells us "Light and darkness are not one, not two."

Zen is quite spare–the main practice is sitting watching the breath.[18] Usually there are no words or visualizations. The practitioner by being aware of the present moment "loses" the small self and participates in the absolute. One can offer a sitting for another person, but there is no sense of holding the image of the person in mind or asking a supreme being for healing or purification. I would call this state "loving intentionality," but others may not agree with me. During Services sutras (scriptures) are chanted, and dedications are read by the lead chanter when the sangha (congregation) prays for resolution of karma:

In reciting the Daihishin Dharani (an incantation) and in offering flowers, candle and incense,
We dedicate its merits to all ancestors of our Zen community members and to all beings in the Dharma worlds.
May penetrating light dispel the darkness of ignorance.
Let all karma be resolved and the mind flower bloom in eternal spring. . . .

or for healing:

We especially pray for the health and well-being of: (names are read)
May they be serene through all their ills
And may we realize the Buddha Way together."

Buddhist funeral services are elaborate and there are food offerings as well as flowers, candle, incense and prayers offered for the one who has died. Devout Japanese Buddhists have a home altar for dead family members and offer daily prayers for them.

THE PROCESS OF PRAYER

So there does seem to be prayer in Buddhism, especially if we are willing to embrace intentionality as the defining factor and if Western religions are willing to accept Dossey's definition of prayer as being "communication with the Absolute" or my own as "becoming one with the Absolute."

The scientific research about the efficacy of prayer in the experiments cited by Dossey, especially those relating to laboratory cultures, is fascinating because the clear implication is: it's not the subject or the object that's paramount, but the process itself. It doesn't seem to matter who is praying, what they are saying (or not saying), for whom or what they are praying, or even more interesting–to whom they are praying. What is important is the general climate created by the prayer. This climate, or sacred space can be achieved by words, music, movement, or silence. This could be problematical for Western theologians because then non-religious psychics might be seen as doing a better job of communicating with the Absolute than ministers, priests or rabbis. Since the Absolute is boundless, those who are able to participate in it sometimes demonstrate supernormal powers–there is a long history of Tibetan Vairayana and Tantric monks being able to sit naked in the snow without freezing or to "float" over the landscape covering miles in a short time.[19] There have always been healers and shamans in tribal cultures. Jesus Christ walked on water and healed the sick. Some people seem to have been born with the ability to touch the Absolute, others have been able to attain it through rigorous practice. Modern Zen practitioners are not encouraged to try to cultivate "magic" or healing powers, but the truth of the matter is that if someone who is participating in the Absolute is praying for me, there might be better results. The Haraldsson and Thorsteinsson paper "Psychokinetic Effects on Yeast" cited by Dossey seems to support my belief. The two spiritual healers and the physician who used spiritual healing and prayer in his practice scored better results than the four students with no experience in healing. When I was a child attending Catholic school we would often pray to the Virgin Mary, asking her to intercede with her Son. If I were ill, I'd be grateful to have the Dalai Lama praying at my bedside–his ability to participate in, to *be* the Absolute is the key point. The Absolute is boundless and an encounter with it creates spaciousness.

As a healthcare chaplain I come into contact with patients and their families who are so paralyzed by pain, fear or anger that their universe has shrunken to a small fist of suffering. I have found that prayer in any form (liturgy, spontaneous prayer, chanting, singing, meditation, visualization) creates a space where constricted energy can be released and open avenues for emotional, spiritual and even physical healing.[20]

When I was a CPE intern, I met an extraordinary Peruvian woman who exuded strength, serenity and equanimity. She had been diagnosed with leukemia when she was 24 years old and had been told she had less than a year to live. When I encountered L., she was 38 years old. She was a devout Catholic who frequently said, "I love my Jesus, He will save me." But her grandmother had been a well-respected shaman and healer in Peru and had taught her (in her own words) "to touch God." L. had worked with a Chi Kung master over the years and attributed her healing to her own spiritual work and to Jesus. Early one morning as I entered her room, I heard her softly singing the sweetest melody in a language I did not recognize. I couldn't bear to interrupt this special moment, but later I asked her about the song and she told me that when she meditated on Jesus she sometimes sang in tongues. From a Buddhist perspective, she was one with the Absolute. Who could not call this prayer? L. had every expectation of leaving the hospital in a few days, and indeed she did.

Quantum Physics is telling us that we are bursts of energy moving so quickly that we only seem to be solid, separate beings. This theory eerily coincides with Buddhist beliefs–there is no solid, separate self–we are all the One Body.[21] Can it be possible that when we are under emotional or physical stress that there is no *space* for healing to take place; no avenues of escape for the viruses and cancers that afflict us? If the flutter of a butterfly's wings in Africa affects our climate in North America, is it possible that the opening of one heart and mind (the one praying) can create space for healing in another? Can I, by participating in the Absolute heal myself? From the Buddhist perspective, the answer is a resounding "Yes."[22]

RECIPROCITY IN PRAYER

If it is the process that's important then the one praying is also receiving benefits. In the Theravada tradition of Buddhism part of the practice called *Metta* meditation *is* to send compassion to another by repeating phrases over and over. The phrases for compassion are:

May you be free from pain.
May you be free from suffering.
May your heart be filled with peace.

One does not attach to the idea of the person being sent *Metta* actually becoming free from suffering. It is our relationship to the other's suffering that is healed and opened up. A space is created where there is no person praying, no person suffering, just unconditional love. It is significant that the alternate phrase taught is:

I care about your pain.

Do we care about pain? So often, as friends and caregivers to those suffering and dying, we erect walls to protect ourselves from becoming overwhelmed by grief. And these protective shields are just what keep us from being totally present to another. Alignment with the Absolute erodes these walls and reveals a space that's serene and wise enough to accept things *as they are,* without the expectation of change. What *is* created, however, is room for the change (or healing) to take place.

Pastoral caregivers often speak about a ministry of presence, and I've noticed that it's not always the dynamic preacher, or the learned theologian, or the experienced minister who is most helpful to patients or family members. Frequently untrained caregivers exhibit a willingness to inhabit the same painful space as the patient, without needing to deny or change anything. The caregiver allows space for things to be as they are. Perhaps we can call this prayerful presence.

When in a hospital room a doctor, nurse, chaplain, and family members are gathered together in communal silence, focusing attention on the patient's well being, it doesn't matter that each person has a different method of praying, or is praying to a different God, or any God at all. The overall effect is that a loving space is being created where healing (medical or otherwise) can enter.

I can see why some fundamentalist religions might recoil at such an idea. For we are not depending on an almighty being outside of ourselves to miraculously heal the sick person. We are simply aligning ourselves with the source of life and trusting that what needs to happen will happen.

PERSONAL IMPLICATIONS OF DOSSEY'S WORK

As a practicing Buddhist I have always been aware of the sacred space that can be created by a person's presence. When one is able to quiet the mind and touch the inner core of non-egoistic equanimity, one is able to act with wisdom and compassion. I know from personal experience that this happens in deep meditation and I believe that it happens in heartfelt prayer or singing or dancing. As a Buddhist chaplain I have been troubled by the prevalent belief among American clergy that communication with the Absolute can be achieved by only certain methods, that there are special words to be said, that there is only one embodiment of the Absolute. I would hope that Dossey's work will encourage some traditionalists to open their minds and hearts to other methods of prayer and to other views of the Absolute.

My own pastoral practice remains the same–I will continue to offer a prayerful presence to those who ask and to train persons in different methods of communicating with the Absolute. I am not particularly excited by the experiments about the power of prayer. America is already a results-driven society. Physical healing is not all there is–spiritual and emotional healing are equally important and how can they be measured? Will a new phenomenon arise, the emergence of expert pray-ers? To me process is important; intention is important; unity with the Absolute is important. Some New Age gurus are telling people that if they get sick it's their own fault. Must we also tell them that if they don't get well it's because they haven't enough faith or their families don't pray hard enough? I've heard that message many times during my work as a chaplain. Sometimes I think we forget that prayer is also to express our gratitude for life, our reverence of the Absolute and unconditional love.

WHAT ROLE WILL PASTORAL CAREGIVERS HAVE IN THIS PROCESS OF INFUSING THE SCIENCE OF MEDICINE WITH THIS NEW SENSE OF SPIRITUALITY?

The reevaluation of the role of pastoral care in clinical settings could be the most important outcome of the scientific research and Dossey's work. Lately the role of chaplains has been undervalued in some clinical settings. It is shown in subtle ways: how doctors may not interact on a collegial level with chaplains and in more blatant ones, for example when chaplains' offices are co-opted by other departments. Frequently pastoral care is seen as a non-billable frill– why keep trained professionals on staff when in a pinch you can always get a local clergyperson to come in when a patient insists?

If it can be demonstrated that prayer or loving intentionality can aid in healing, shorten recovery times, lower blood pressure and relieve stress so that less anesthesia is needed, and reduce recurrence of disease, then the role of a pastoral caregiver has value in the money-driven world of big business hospitals. This is just a superficial change.

The real revolution can be that pastoral caregivers will be used more as part of the surgical team, work in concert with pain management, work with families and friends in order to create a healing environment and train healthcare professionals in "communicating with the Absolute" while they work. There is a famous Zen koan:

A monk asked, "What is Zen?"
The master replied, "Chopping wood, carrying water."

When one experiences work (whatever it is) as prayer, life is never the same. Each moment, each gesture, each word is fresh. We recreate ourselves in each moment and so are able to give of ourselves freely, never fearing that we'll run out of resources. We can act with wisdom and compassion and then let go.

AUTHOR NOTE

Madeline Ko-i Bastis, a Zen priest and board-certified chaplain, is the founder and director of Peaceful Dwelling Project, Inc., 2 Harbourview Drive, East Hampton, NY 11937 (e-mail: peacefuldwell~hamptons.com). This is a non-profit foundation that offers pastoral care to patients and staffs outside the hospital environment by facilitating nondenominational retreats where persons with life-challenging illness and professional caregivers can communicate with the Absolute in a variety of ways–prayer, meditation, visualization, music, writing and movement in order to heal themselves and others. PDP also trains healthcare professionals and clergy from different traditions in using meditation/visualization for spiritual, emotional and physical healing.

REFERENCES

1. Walpola Rahula. *What the Buddha Taught* (New York: Grove Weidenfeld, 1959).
2. Rahula, 16.
3. Philip Kapleau. *The Three Pillars of Zen* (New York: Anchor Doubleday, 1989), 38.
4. Joseph Goldstein and Jack Kornfeld. *Seeking the Heart of Wisdom: the Path of Insight Meditation* (Boston: Shambala, 1988).
5. Paul Williams. *Mahayana Buddhism: The Doctrinal Foundations* (London: Routledge, 1989).
6. Sharon Salzberg. *Loving-Kindness: The Revolutionary Art of Happiness* (Boston: Shambala, 1995).

7. Nyanaponika Thera. "Karma and its fruit" in S. Bercholz and T. Kohn, (eds.) *Entering the Stream: An Introduction to the Buddha and His Teachings* (Shambala: Boston, 1993), 122-129.

8. K. Tanaka. *The Dawn of Chinese Pure Land Buddhist Doctrine* (Albany: SUNY, 1990).

9. Paul Swanson. *Foundations of T'ien T'ai Philosophy* (Berkeley: Asian Humanities Press,1989).

10. Taiko Yamasaki. *Shingon: Japanese Esoteric Buddhism* (Boston: Shambala, 1988).

11. Sandy McIntosh. "As American as apple pie? An insiders view of Nichiren Shoshu" In *Tricycle: the Buddhist Review* Winter, 1992 18-25.

12. McIntosh, 22.

13. McIntosh, 23.

14. Sogyal Rinpoche. *The Tibetan Book of Living and Dying* (San Francisco: Harper Collins, 1992), 240.

15. John Powers. *Introduction to Tibetan Buddhism* (Ithaca: Snow Lion, 1995), 145.

16. Sogyal Rinpoche, 313.

17. Pema Chodron. *The Wisdom of No Escape* (Boston: Shambala, 1991), 56-64.

18. Shunryu Suzuki. *Zen Mind, Beginner's Mind* (New York: Weatherill, 1970), 29-31.

19. Lama Govinda. *Foundations of Tibetan Mysticism* (London: Rider, 1959), 172.

20. Sogyal Rinpoche, 41-55.

21. Philip Kapleau, 61-63.

22. Stephen Levine. *Who Dies?–An Investigation of Conscious Living and Conscious Dying* (New York: Anchor Books, 1982).

A Response to Larry Dossey:
Prayer, Medicine, and Science:
The New Dialogue

David C. Baker, PhD, BCC

Writing a response to Larry Dossey's article has forced me to revisit a number of my own assumptions and beliefs about intercessory prayer, and to stretch my understanding of the nature of prayer and how it functions. The scientist within me was pleased to know that there is empirical support for the efficaciousness of what I have been doing myself and encouraging others to do for years. *I initially welcomed his challenge to take prayer seriously, but as I examined my faith and pastoral practice, I was reminded of the difficulty of discerning what to pray for and the enduring problem of unanswered prayer.* While intercessory prayer has been a part of the Judeo-Christian culture and practice since its beginning, the dilemma remains about how one is to deal with these nagging questions. Let me share a recent personal example.

After waiting a long while for a donor, a colleague of my wife underwent transplant surgery. When I learned of the occasion of her

David C. Baker is Director of Chaplaincy Services, LAS Passavant Retirement Community, Zelienople, PA 16063.

[Haworth co-indexing entry note]: "A Response to Larry Dossey: Prayer, Medicine, and Science: The New Dialogue." Baker, David C. Co-published simultaneously in *Journal of Health Care Chaplaincy* (The Haworth Pastoral Press, an imprint of The Haworth Press, Inc.) Vol. 7, No. 1/2, 1998, pp. 97-104; and: *Scientific and Pastoral Perspectives on Intercessory Prayer: An Exchange Between Larry Dossey, M.D. and Health Care Chaplains* (ed: Larry VandeCreek) The Haworth Pastoral Press, an imprint of The Haworth Press, Inc., 1998, pp. 97-104; and: *Scientific and Pastoral Perspectives on Intercessory Prayer: An Exchange Between Larry Dossey, M.D. and Health Care Chaplains* (ed: Larry VandeCreek) Harrington Park Press, an imprint of The Haworth Press, Inc., 1998, pp. 97-104. Single or multiple copies of this article are available for a fee from The Haworth Document Delivery Service [1-800-342-9678, 9:00 a.m. - 5:00 p.m. (EST). E-mail address: getinfo@haworth.com].

surgery, I immediately offered a silent prayer asking God that her procedure go well and that she fully recover. Last month, exactly one year later from the day of the surgery, she had to have the same procedure repeated because her body had rejected the first donated organ. And like last year, once again, when I learned of her surgery, I offered a brief silent prayer that all would go well and that, this time, it would "take." Would my prayer be efficacious? Based on the "failure" of the first transplant, was my first prayer efficacious? Did it fall on deaf ears? Was there something wrong or lacking in my prayer? Were enough people praying for the patient? What exactly happened last year? And what will happen this year? Fortunately for the patient, at the time of this writing, the second surgery seems to have been successful and the rejection problems manageable.

I serve in a continuing care retirement community with persons who experience chronic illness, major losses, and critical changes in their health and lifestyle. When asked to pray for them, I often find myself not wanting to pray that a miracle take place that would restore their physical health or circumstance, but that they be granted the courage and strength to accept the things that have occurred. Is this a lack of faith in the power of prayer on my part? Or is it an expression of my modern world view about how God operates in the universe? I am not alone on this issue, for already a century ago, Sören Kierkegaard held that to believe that God acts on human beings in an external way is superstition. For him, God acts only on human inwardness; the efficacy of prayer lies in the inner transformation of the one who prays. According to Kierkegaard, prayer is something we do so that God can do something to us so that we can see ourselves honestly as we are and thereby be transformed more into God's image. Prayer is a matter of discerning how God's healing activity is manifesting itself in our lives at a particular time.[1]

But I wonder, is this limiting the power of prayer? Is my reluctance to pray for miracles a lack of faith shaped my own cultural world view? In earlier times when science was limited and prayer was seen as petitioning God for special favors, it was understood that God could and did intervene in the history and lives of people. However, in a modern time of great science and technology, intercessory prayer and supernatural intervention seem inessential and non-existent to many, including faithful Christian pastors and chaplains. Recently, one Sunday at worship, I was asked to pray for rain because it had been rather warm and dry lately and the local yards and gardens were suffering. I did so, even though the weather forecast was indicating that we would likely experience rain later that day, which we did. I wonder, "Was my prayer necessary? Whom did it serve?"

Our metaphors and language determine how we understand God. In a modern world, one wonders if the traditional construct of God being a personal being with whom we can dialogue is still valid, or must we seek new models for our understanding of prayer? Dossey believes that unless we learn to see the world in new ways, we shall remain unable to engage the evidence on intercessory prayer. He states that people deny the efficaciousness of prayer, not because of insufficient empirical evidence, but rather from a failure of imagination. "Unable to see how prayer could work, too many people insist that it cannot work." He concludes that a new paradigm is needed, and suggests that the language of parapsychology and the metaphor of distant mental phenomena may be the answer.

While I appreciate Dossey's effort to reach those who are struggling with prayer, from the perspective of Christian faith, we do not need another paradigm—we already have one that works. What we need is a renewal of faith because prayer is rooted in trust. We are invited to pray believing that our prayers are heard and responded to by a loving "heavenly Father." The outcome may or may not be as we ask, but, in faith, we trust that God hears our petitions and is acting in the best interest of the recipient of the prayer. "Faith defies logic and propels us beyond hope. . . . It allows us to live by the grace of invisible strands. It is a belief in a wisdom superior to our own."[2] At the same time, if prayer is an expression of faith, then it is ultimately dependent on God's action, for St. Paul tells us that faith is a gift from God.[3] The initiative which moves a person to pray or to struggle with the whole concept of prayer is God's.

Prayer is an expression of our deepest being. It is that which distinguishes living faith from a purely intellectual view of the world and from philosophical interpretations of human nature and destiny. The assumption about prayer is that it presupposes a responsiveness in the Divine, and assumes that God is friendly, trust-worthy, and dependable. Following the example and teachings of Jesus, the early Church prayed for specific needs of others, often repeatedly, and always with the notion of ultimately committing the situation to God.[4] It was not understood as a magical manipulation of God but rather an expression of the living relationship in which creatures relate to their Creator. Jesus, when instructing his disciples how to pray, addressed the Creator in very personal terms, inferring that we can approach the Creator as little children making our needs known to a gracious, loving Father.[5]

If one believes in the efficaciousness of intercessory prayer, then one must wrestle with the matter of determining to what end the intercessory prayer resource should be used. This would seem to pose an ethical issue of what to pray for and whose will should be done. Whose needs or intentions are more honorable or worthy of intercessory prayer? Do we pray to destroy the microbiology of a disease, or do we pray that a harmonious balance can occur that allows all living organisms to co-exist? By praying to remedy one problem, do we create or allow another problem to impact our world? Since everything is ecologically linked, how do we know what to pray to change? In the Lord's Prayer, Jesus asks for specif-ics–daily bread, to not be led into temptation, and so on, yet before asking for anything, Jesus asks that God's will be done on earth as in heaven.[6] He teaches us that we should both ask for what we need and yet maintain an openness to accept whatever happens as part of God's divine providence. At the same time, we can find comfort in St. Paul's words, who teaches that the Holy Spirit knows the mind of God and is therefore able to shape our prayers in accordance with divine purpose.[7]

Dossey cites several studies whose data suggest that intercessory prayer works although how it works is not clear. He points out that science often is able to demonstrate empirical facts long before it can develop an acceptable theory to explain the phenomena. Some would say that it is just a matter of time for science to explore and understand the means of intercessory prayer, while others believe that it may never be understood. Like the nature of God, Himself, its mechanism may lay beyond the reach of words and concepts. For me, the mechanics of prayer is a moot issue. I know that intercessory prayer works because I have witnessed it enable people to find peace in impossible circumstances. It is successful, not because it can be demonstrated rationally, but because it is effective in preventing despair and inspiring hope. I have seen it in those I have ministered to, and I have experienced its power myself. It reminds me of that television pain-reliever commercial where the speaker confides that when he is looking for a solution to his headache, he does not depend on the results of clinical studies but rather on what brand of medicine his doctor actually uses.

I agree whole-heartedly with Dossey that we need not suspend our belief in prayer nor deny the evidence of it while we wait for an adequate scientific explanation. For me, the mechanics of intercessory prayer are merely another mystery of the Transcendent. I do not always understand the internal workings of the computer system with which I am constructing this essay, but I know how to utilize the few basic commands I have been taught, and as I follow my instructions, in faith I trust that I will be able to generate a product.

I am uncomfortable with Dossey's lumping together of distant mental phenomena of parapsychology and intercessory prayer. While they may both begin in the mind, the distant mental phenomena clearly appears to be a human effort, while the intercessory prayer, by Western definition, requires a distant agent to produce the desired effect. I take delight in Dossey's depiction of God in heaven acting as a kind of "satellite" waiting for believers to send a prayer request so that He might relay that request into an effective "outcome" for the intended recipient. This concept is more comfortable for me to believe and to apply in my pastoral practice. It also seems to be shared by everyone with whom I work.

At the same time, I must admit that this model does not fit other cultures where God is not understood as a distant "Other" or "personal," and I am not sure how to resolve this problem. Dossey may be right when he suggests that intercessory prayer may really be a distant mental phenomena whereby we somehow consciously and intentionally effect change in the physical world by our generating some form of mental energy. Dossey cites evidence from the field of physics that would seem to support this possibility. Perhaps all consciousness is somehow linked both with itself and with non-conscious matter, and therefore we are able to alter the object of our attention. Who is to say that this was not the means by which Jesus was able to perform his healing miracles? Was he able to intensely focus or direct his inner resources or somehow harness some external power of God to accomplish what he did? Scripture informs us that Jesus had a kind of power (τηνδυναμιν) that was described as a physical emanation coming from him that healed people who came into contact with him.[8] Did not the crowds often push upon him in order to touch him?[9] Did he not often physically touch those whom he healed or raised from the dead? Was not the woman with a long-time hemorrhage healed merely by touching his robe, and was not Jesus aware that "power" had gone from him?[10] Jesus empowered and sent his disciples out on a mission to heal the sick and raise the dead.[11] The early Church practiced prayer and healing, and included belief in the "laying on of hands" as an important part of early doctrine.[12] Has the Church, two thousand years later, somehow lost some critical components of the faith–perhaps some of the things that Jesus in his great commission may have been referring to when he instructed his disciples to teach all that he had commanded them? As St. Paul tells us, we see as in a mirror dimly. Hopefully someday, we'll understand in full.

Dossey proposes that subjects in studies of distant intentionality use a kind of "wordless beseeching" by which they try to coax, nudge or somehow help the experiment toward a certain outcome, much as one does when one tries to guide a car along an icy road or perform any exacting piece of work under all but impossible situations. Dossey suggests that such "beseeching" is a kind of "prayer." Perhaps there is more to what St. Paul meant when he spoke of prayer in terms of the Spirit groaning within us.[13] Dossey states that such "beseeching" is used by many people in their daily business as they express empathy and care for others. It is yet a mystery, and Dossey says, we will need a new model to more fully explain the phenomenon.

However it operates, prayer is an integral part of pastoral ministry. As a representative of the Christ and his Church, a chaplain or pastor embodies the presence of the Divine in the context of human need. When making a pastoral visit, I demonstrate pastoral care through my presence and through my active listening, and after seeking to understand the person's concerns, I customarily offer to pray for the person as a way of helping the person to summarize his or her concerns and articulate them to God.

When the person asks for miraculous healing, however, I must admit that, as I speak the words of prayer, sometimes I am skeptical whether God will answer their request as they make it. Yet, in obedience to our Lord's invitation to pray, and in support of the one making the request, I offer the prayer on their behalf as a way of providing hope at a time when that person's life is in great distress. I am their advocate to the One who can transform them. God may or may not choose to do so as I ask, but nevertheless, He will touch them. While some may question whether this is being honest, my pastoral calling is to walk with persons through their valley of the shadow, assisting them to engage the Eternal in meaningful ways that enable them to successfully face their problems. By joining with the person in the midst of their need, I can establish a relationship that will permit me to accompany the person on a journey that may involve his or her having to accept the givens of their situation.

A primary purpose of intercessory prayer is to facilitate healing of mind, body, and spirit. While it may involve physical healing, intercessory prayer can also provide an exercise in faith which can support one's search for meaning in the midst of suffering and pain. It can remind one of his or her identity as being a beloved child of God. It can enable one to be calm in the midst of highly stressful situations.

For those who wish to better utilize prayer as a resource for medical intervention and other applications, it would seem logical to continue to research it, teasing out what knowledge and understanding one can. Whatever that outcome, chaplains and pastors currently possess a valuable resource to employ for the comfort and care of those we serve. Dossey is right when he says that prayer does not need science to validate it. People use it daily, and know its power, so let us not waste it while we debate its attributes or mechanism. After all, as human beings, all we can ever hope to understand about prayer is the human side of our dialogue with God. Because He is beyond our comprehension, we cannot fathom how God hears or responds to the prayer.

Those of us who are employed in the health care field as spiritual caregivers must begin to raise consciousness of the efficacy of prayer both among ourselves and among those other health care professionals with whom we work. We must be engaging the whole medical system to inform it that prayer works and that spiritual care is a vital component of wholistic care. In times of health care reform and managed care with limited and shrinking resources for medical intervention, the intentional use of prayer to assist in bringing about healing would seem especially prudent.

REFERENCES

1. Edward P. Wimberly. *Pastoral Care in the Black Church* (Nashville: Abingdon Press, 1979), 14.

2. Terry T. Williams. *Refuge: An Unnatural History of Family and Place* (New York: Vantage Books, 1991), 198.

3. Ephesians 2:8.

4. Matthew 6:33; Luke 6:28; John 17:9; Colossians 1:9; James 5:16; I Thessalonians 5:17.

5. Matthew 7:7-9.

6. Matthew 6:9-13.

7. Romans 8:26ff.

8. Luke 6:19.

9. Mark 3:10.

10. Mark 5:25-32.

11. Matthew 10:1-10.

12. Hebrews 6:2.

13. Romans 8:26.

Response to Larry Dossey:
Prayer, Medicine, and Science:
The New Dialogue

Patricia Swanson Megregian, MDiv, BCC

I first heard Dr. Larry Dossey speak in 1995 at a conference in Buffalo, New York. He presented his topic on the power of intercessory prayer to a group of health care providers, hospice care givers, nurses, doctors, social workers, and clergy. His message claiming the power of intercessory prayer to help in care of patients was captivating. It was intriguing because it came from the very profession that has so long separated itself from any kind of public acknowledgement of the impact of a person's spiritual life on health and healing. As he described his experiences in his clinical practice and the results of research into intercessory prayer, I remember leaning over to my colleague attending with me saying, "This feels like home to me." This I had experienced. This I have known.

At the heart of Dr. Larry Dossey's message is an experience that changed how he cared for his patients as a physician, as a scientist, and as a fellow human being. I understand his goal to be sharing

Patricia Swanson Megregian is Director of Spiritual Care, Children's Hospital, Buffalo, NY 14222.

[Haworth co-indexing entry note]: "Response to Larry Dossey: Prayer, Medicine, and Science: The New Dialogue." Megregian, Patricia Swanson. Co-published simultaneously in *Journal of Health Care Chaplaincy* (The Haworth Pastoral Press, an imprint of The Haworth Press, Inc.) Vol. 7, No. 1/2, 1998, pp. 105-116; and: *Scientific and Pastoral Perspectives on Intercessory Prayer: An Exchange Between Larry Dossey, M.D. and Health Care Chaplains* (ed: Larry VandeCreek) The Haworth Pastoral Press, an imprint of The Haworth Press, Inc., 1998, pp. 105-116; and: *Scientific and Pastoral Perspectives on Intercessory Prayer: An Exchange Between Larry Dossey, M.D. and Health Care Chaplains* (ed: Larry VandeCreek) Harrington Park Press, an imprint of The Haworth Press, Inc., 1998, pp. 105-116. Single or multiple copies of this article are available for a fee from The Haworth Document Delivery Service [1-800-342-9678, 9:00 a.m. - 5:00 p.m. (EST). E-mail address: getinfo@haworth.com].

that experience with others in the health care field, especially other physicians, whether by means of repetition of the experience in scientific research or supporting that experience in religious tradition. What is ground breaking is that he is a physician who openly practices intercessory prayer as a healing modality along with surgery or drugs. For that alone, we as chaplains should applaud his work.

Dr. Dossey gives chaplains an entrance into the world of medicine through the discipline of laboratory research and study that has thus far been the domain of research scientists and academic physicians. He is calling for chaplains to join in the search for how this phenomena of intercessory prayer—or non-local intention—works to benefit the very patients we serve.

My own attempt to try and incorporate complimentary therapies—such as meditation, relaxation techniques and energy work into spiritual care—was met with my Vice-President of Nursing saying, "I'm supportive of trying new things and this sounds like a good idea. After all, the public is going to want these services but we have to do outcome studies." And, she was correct in encouraging me to do the research needed. Interestingly, traditional prayer is an accepted practice in the hospital. It always has been. Is it because the health care workers view it as comforting, but hardly powerful enough to make a difference on the physical outcome of the patient? *Most often, we as chaplains are called in by the physicians at the end of life when there are no more procedures left to do, or the situation is beyond the control of the physicians to save a patient's life. What Dr. Dossey proposes is that intercessory prayer be used at the very onset of treatment.* However, if that was really done, it would mean a paradigm shift in the way physicians and health care workers think about prayer.

I have become convinced since I have been working in a hospital that anyone—whether it is a physician, scientist, chaplain, patient, or family member—must first experience the connection with the Holy in some way. The experience must come first. It could be on a mountain top or in a test tube. But, one must first have the "AH HA" moment before one can ever set out on the journey of discovery. One must be able to experience the power of intercessory prayer, the phenomena of parapsychology, or the results of non-local intention in order to even want to seek understanding or make it a part of care for others. Talking about it is one thing, experiencing it is another. Once you have experienced the Mystery, it becomes a part of your life. That is where the journey must begin for all of us.

There is a wonderful book called, *Belonging to the Universe: Explorations on the Frontiers of Science & Spirituality* which is a dialogue between Fritjof Capra, Ph.D., author of *The Tao of Physics* and David Steindl-Rast, Ph.D., a Benedictine monk. These two are described on the cover of the book as, "The trailblazer in new science and a contemporary Thomas Merton investigates the parallels between new paradigm thinking in science and religion, which together offer a remarkably compatible new view of the universe." The book is in dialogue form and they are talking about science and theology.

> Fritjof: I think of the image of a wave, which you like to use, David, is a very apt one. The theologian and the scientist are like two corks floating on the same wave. The wave would be the collective consciousness, the culture, or the Zeitgeist, something like this. This collective consciousness is going through a change of paradigms, a groundswell, as it were. I think that is the common ground. It manifests itself in science, and it manifests itself in theology. . . .[1]

They go on to talk about the similarities of science and theology.

> Fritjof: The similarities are that both are based on experience and on a certain kind of systematic observation, so they are empirical. Of course, there are great differences in the way scientists observe. But our disciplines are both theoretical reflections on experience.[1]

After reading Dr. Dossey's article, I was reminded of the importance of the intention in those experiences we have whether we are praying with a patient and family or praying for bacteria to grow. I must constantly be asking questions of myself. Do I have compassion for this child? Am I treating this person in a non-judgmental way? Do I, in fact, love them? My participation in the moment of intercessory prayer is crucial to the power of the prayer. That is the responsibility we accept as participants in the Mystery of life.

One of the recent experiences I had in the ICU was in fact, life changing for me. It was 2:00 A.M. when the telephone woke me up from a deep sleep. It was the ICU wanting me to come into the hospital to say a prayer for a dying child. When I arrived, the nurse explained that the patient was an 18 year old boy who had a congenital syndrome that caused his body to grow more and more deformed but that his mind was normal.

He had complications from surgery and now his body was filled with infection. His organs were shutting down and the ICU physician had done everything that was possible and they were losing the fight. The physicians had given him only a couple hours longer to live. He was sedated and quiet. His mother was at his side holding his hand and weeping. I introduced myself as the chaplain and told her how sorry I was that he was so sick. She confirmed what the doctors had told me about his condition but quickly told me she still believed that he could somehow survive by some miracle.

I sat with her for awhile talking softly about his life, about his dreams, looking at pictures of the senior prom which he had been able to attend recently. In the intimacy of the moment, I asked her if she wanted to pray together. She said yes, please. I placed one hand on the child's forehead, the other was holding his hand. I recalled the ancient tradition of the laying on of hands for the sick and dying as I closed my eyes to pray. Ordinarily, I would have begun my prayer that God be present in this difficult time for the child and for the mother even though I knew at the same time Mom would be praying for a miracle cure.

But that night, in the quiet of the humming machines and the shadows of the late night death watch, I was led to pray something entirely different. I prayed that God's golden light of love come into the child and literally push the infection out of his body. I asked for him to be completely filled with God. Suddenly, I felt my hands grow warm. They started to tingle. I felt as if I were a vessel being filled with God's love and pouring that love into this child. I was awed, frightened, and curious about this strange experience.

I quickly looked at his mother to see what affect this might have had on her. Did she sense anything different than the usual prayers given at the bedside? She had her head bowed and her eyes closed. I ended the prayer asking for God to do what was the very best for this child and we would wait and listen for the answer. I walked out of the room and slumped against the wall. The nurse came over with concern in her eyes. "Are you all right?" she said.

"Yes," I said. "*Something strange happened in there, though. I'm not sure what it was but I just laid hands on that boy and prayed for him to be healed even though I have been told he is going to die soon. Listen,*" I stuttered, "*something happened to my hands when I was praying. I felt a great power come through me.*"

"*Jeez!*" she said, "*You're scaring me. I've got goose bumps on my arms.*"

"Look," I whispered, "It could be nothing so don't say anything to anyone." But, I know something happened in there. Two hours went by and the boy was still the same. I asked the nurse to call me when there was a change.

I never got called. I went in the next morning to find that he had pulled through the night against all odds and it looked like they were beginning to win the battle with the infection. One month later, he was getting ready to leave the hospital to go for rehabilitation and I stopped by to say goodbye.

"You know," I said, "You are my miracle boy."

He smiled at me with tears in his eyes, "I know. Thank you so much. Will you pray with me before I leave?"

And we did.

In this experience, it all came together. I prayed with the intention of great love for that child. We connected with the power of the Holy and the outcome was a healing of his body. The outcome could have been different. Yet, it would not have negated the experience nor the connection. From that experience, I was led to the study of Reiki, a Japanese laying on of hands healing modality using God's universal energy for the benefit of the patient. Outcome studies of this form of intercessory prayer are in the planning stage and it is now being offered as one of the services the Department of Spiritual Care offers along with prayer, sacraments, worship, meditation and relaxation.

Dr. Larry Dossey has given both physicians and chaplains permission to go beyond the boundaries in which tradition has placed us to reclaim the power our patients need for healing. Physicians have cured the body without taking into account the soul and clergy have worked with the Spirit so long they have forgotten how to bring it back to the soul. It is in the soul where body and spirit come together for healing. The physician and the chaplain are two halves of one whole.

Knowing that Dr. Dossey and others are already reaching for new understandings into intercessory prayer, non-local phenomena, and parapsychology gives me and others the freedom and the forum to join in the quest for increased understanding. After all, at the center of the quest for all of us is the hope that all God's creation will be helped and healed. Because of my experiences in the hospital, because of physicians like Dr. Dossey, the journey to bring together the Mystery of the Holy and the practical life of medicine and healing has begun. It is grounding the spirit into the body. This is not new but ancient. What is new, is our scientific ability to measure and test results. The chaplain and the physician are natural partners in that journey.

Later in the book, *Belonging to the Universe . . . ,* the dialog reflects on this topic.

> David: Now, you are certainly not saying that science and theology are concerned with two different realms of reality but with one and the same realm from different aspects. Is that correct?
>
> Fritjof: First of all, I would say they are both concerned with human experience . . . Science asks for the how and theology, the why. I agree with that. But then the how and the why can not always be separated. Science asks for the how, more precisely for how a particular phenomenon is connected to all the other phenomena. If you include more and more connections, ultimately you will reveal the entire context, which is, in fact, the why. Why is connected with meaning, if you are defining meaning as context.[1]

What a creative partnership! The scientist asks how and the chaplain seeks to find meaning. We both have our own perspective, yet we both seek the Truth. I do believe that Dr. Dossey's answer to "how" does lie in the new quantum thinking of physics. Since the discovery of quantum mechanics and Einstein's theory of relativity, all facets of our culture and experience, including theology, have responded to this new paradigm thinking.

I am a practical life theologian. I understand that the most important thing in life is connections and experiences. It is our interaction with people, with the world, and with God that ultimately count for our time on earth. This concept of connections emphasized by quantum physics helps me focus my ministry. When I know that no matter what occurs or with whom it occurs, all that happens is within God, I can help people cope with a world that appears out of control. Things happen to people. Some are a product of their own decisions or the result of someone else's decision but there are things that happen to people out of their control. They just happen. Some would say that particles of energy come together and make a connection. It is as simple as that. But, what you do in the situation is what really counts.

Rabbi Edwin Friedman spoke in a wonderful video taped from the Alban Institute called, *Family Process and Process Theology:*

> Life is a process of events, a string of occasions, an ever changing progression. That is reality. What is permanent, what continues is relationships, connections, patterns that are passed down from one generation to another. It is not substance that is permanent but the way things come together. Every event is an inheritor of things in the past. Cumulative secession is the real nature of life.[2]

The search for our interconnectedness is unending. It is the stuff of the universe. It is the essence of God. We are all participants in a constantly changing cosmos and what we do and say makes a difference to those around us both near and far. Thomas Matus a member of the dialogue team in *Belonging to the Universe* connect the physician and the chaplain this way:

> It seems to me that you have hit upon the point where the new paradigms in science and theology converge: the realization that the 'objective viewpoint' is illusory, that in the face of total reality, no one can be a 'detached observer.' . . . It is your story that is being told, you are part of it all. So the shift from the part to the whole also involves the realization that I belong

> to the whole universe, not as if I were a negligible phenome-
> non on a small planet in a minor solar system but as a vital
> participation in the living cosmos. This realization is both the
> context and the condition of God's self-disclosure.[1]

It is this participation in the universe that gives us permission to
seek the laboratory and ask God to disclose our universe.

As a chaplain, I am always searching for meaning in the traumas
and tragedies I experience every day in the hospital. I have found
the work of philosopher and theologian, Charles Hartshorne, who
developed "Process Theology" to be extremely challenging and
helpful. I consider him to be a new paradigm thinker. My continuing understanding of Hartshorne's philosophy comes from a colleague and friend, Rev. Dr. Ralph Carnes, Ph.D. a Board Certified
Chaplain and student of Hartshorne, with whom I have had a professional dialogue concerning these concepts for years.

Hartshorne understands God as panentheistic. That is, God is a
person, but a person that is made up of all that is and has been, and
who is, in some way conscious of being a person, an entity. This is a
different understanding than the oriental pantheists found in eastern
religions, where God is the universe, is everything, in everything,
and does not have consciousness of an entity separate from the
universe. For Hartshorne, the universe is part of God in the same
way that our bodies are a part of us. *If my own body made up of
molecules can be conscious as a self, then how much greater is
God's awareness that S/He is God, God who is made up of all the
protons, neutrons, leptons, pions, comets, planets, stars, and galax-
ies.*

But God is not simply the sum total of the physical universe with
some consciousness of being the universe. For Hartshorne, all of
history is made up of events, experiences or connections that come
from the subatomic particles all the way up to the level of the mind
of God. So God is made up of all these experiences, which in
process theology is the universe. It is more than matter. It is experience as well.

Hartshorne understood that the process of events and experiences
is what is real. It is not the unchanging substance that is real but the
process of events that is reality. Within the process, human beings,

as part of God, experience the universe from their own unique perspective. Everything that they experience in their lives is never lost but held in God forever. When we die, in fact, we are never lost because all of our experiences are forever in God.

Prayer, then, is an experience that is never lost but is held forever in the mind of God. There is a book recommended to me called, *The Philosophy of Charles Hartshorn,* which consists of essays by various philosophers about Hartshorne's philosophy, and is then answered by the philosopher, himself. In the book, there is an essay by William Reese, "The Trouble with Panentheism" which addresses the concept of panentheism and prayer. Hartshorne responds to Reese in the following way:

> When Reese writes that in perception we do not intuit as obvious the awareness of other persons or of the universe, and that "philosophers agree we lack direct awareness of other minds," I am a little troubled. Whitehead and I hold that in all experience there is "feeling of feeling," where the second token of the word refers to feelings whose feelers are other actual entities. And some of these other actual feelers are not members of the sequence of actual entities forming one's own stream of awareness. So there is direct awareness of other minds. One intuits, I hold, the pleasant and unpleasant feelings of one's own bodily cells. They, in their vastly inferior fashion, feel our feelings, and analogously, we feel God's feelings; and God in vastly, indeed ideally, superior fashion feels ours.[3]

Intercessory prayer, then, is one person experiencing the love and compassion for another person within God. When we talk to each other, we also talk to God. When we talk to God, we also talk to each other. As we both live in God, we both live together. When we are both dead, we will both still live in God. But our awareness will join God's awareness. God feels our feelings, as we feel God. So, there is no "apartness," either from each other or from God. The "apartness" that we feel is only an illusion. There is no life outside of God.

Hartshorne's God which includes the universe, is made up of spirit or mind. That is why it is sometimes referred to as "pansychism," which is the theory that there is no matter in the universe, just mind. For Hartshorne, reality itself is mind; but when it comes to God, "mind" means so much more than the medical terminology means when applied to human beings.

If the scientist asks the question, "does intercessory prayer, parapsychology and non-local phenomena work and if so, how?" and researches that in the laboratory, then the other member of the team, the chaplain can ask the question, "why." It is in Hartshorne's concept of panentheism that we may find direction for answering "why." I find this theology one that works in my day-to-day work with children and families.

My call to the Pediatric Intensive Care Unit was for T., a child that I had been seeing on a continuing basis. He had been admitted the night before with complications from his brain tumor which had been diagnosed at age one month. Now at 10 months old, he had been through the rigors of surgery, chemotherapy, and finally radiation. All the therapies had helped to some extent, but T. still had some remains of his tumor and the side affects of the intensive therapies. In the past, I had always offered a supporting presence and prayers as they walked their difficult journey as a family.

His mother was a quiet, shy woman, who loved her son desperately but often felt overwhelmed by the medical establishment in which she found herself emersed. When I saw her that night, she had tears in her eyes. She held out her hands to me and said, "Everyone has given up on T. Do you think he is going to die?"

I hugged her and sat down. "I don't know. I hope not," I said. "What do you feel? What does your heart tell you?"

She got a determined look in her eye, "I haven't given up on him. He is my son. Everyone else can give up on him but I won't. I'm all he has to fight for him."

She continued, "I called the priest to come and pray for him. He is known to be a healer. He prayed for him right after he had his radiation. When they took the MRI, the tumor had really gotten smaller. I think it was because of the priest's prayers."

I held her hand. And then she asked an unexpected question.

"Why do some people have the gift of healing? What is it that happens when they pray?"

I took a deep breath and paused. I realized what I was going to say was something I certainly would not have said a few years ago.

When I visited the patient, I had just come from reading Dr. Larry Dossey's article for the third time. Did I really believe that prayer worked or had I too fallen into the abyss of too many babies and children dying, too many grief stricken parents, and too many desperate prayers seemingly unanswered. Do I really believe that what I say and do makes a difference? What DID that priest do?

So, I said, "Let me think a minute how to answer you." And I took those minutes to ask for some guidance. This is what I did say to her. "What I think is that all things are connected to each other and that God is in all things including you and me and T. *When a healer prays, he or she makes some kind of intentional connection, taps into God as the Great Healer, the One who loves and wants that best for each one of us, the universal energy of Love that is around us and in us and through us and directs that energy into the person they are praying for.* This great Love is an amazing power. If it is the best thing for T. to be healed, he will be. One thing you need to know is that you also have that connection to God and to T. as much as the priest does. The love you have for him is the same love that God has for him. When you pray, pray directly to the Spirit of God that is inside T. Lay your hands on his head and just love him. Pour that love into him as if it were liquid gold. Surround him with your love knowing that when you do, God's love is also surrounding him. Spend time just laying your hands and meditating how much he is loved."

A few weeks later I saw her up on the floor. Things eased up a bit and he was stable for the moment. She thanked me for talking with her and said that every time she lay hands on T.'s head to pray for him, he would reach up and hold her hands. He wouldn't let her go but seemed to love the feeling of her hands on his head. She also experienced a peace that helped her get through his rough moments. Is it the power of intercessory prayer? The power of love? God's energy? How does it work? It is a mystery which hopefully, someday, we will understand better. My hunch is that as we discover how things work, we will only be brought to another mystery. It is the process of connections that moves us into more understanding. Will we ever know it all? I don't thing so.

The most important element, however, is connections. My response to Dr. Dossey's article is to become connected to my physi-

cian colleagues who are interested in seeking more understanding and scientific knowledge into the mystery of intercessory prayer. Remembering that nothing is outside of God, we are able to ask important questions of parapsychology and quantum theories of non-local phenomena without feeling threatened or being on the fringes of faith. Our goal is to work as a team to explore the ever changing and ever expanding mind of God. At the heart of the universe is the heart of God and that is the ultimate connection for the chaplain, the scientist, and the patient.

REFERENCES

1. Fritjof Capra & David Steindl-Rast. *Belonging to the Universe* (Harper San-Francisco, 1991), 18-19, 161.

2. Edwin H., Friedman. *Family Process and Process Theology* (Washington DC: The Alban Institute, Inc., 1991) Video.

3. L. E. Hahn (ed). *The Philosophy of Charles Hartshorne* (LaSalle, Illinois: Open Court, 1991).

Considering the Dangers
and Opportunities
of Pastoral Care and Medicine:
A Search for Vitality, Accountability
and Balance

Rhoda Toperzer, MDiv

The Chinese word for "crisis" consists of two characters "opportunity" and "danger." Dossey's contribution in the lead article represents both for the pastoral care profession. I believe that his work presents much more "opportunity" than "danger," but both are present. That is the essence of my response; my additional comments elaborate these two themes.

Crises can often be prevented by early accurate assessment of a situation and proactive responses. *The ground may be breaking open for major paradigm shifts, both in spiritual communities and individual lives of faith. The burgeoning interest in spirituality contrasts with an ongoing decline in participation and membership in religious communities.* Opportunity, as well as danger, can hide in the chasm between people's expressed needs and what religious leaders offer in response to those expressed needs. It remains to be

Rhoda Toperzer is Chaplain, Department of Pastoral Care, The Ohio State University Medical Center, Columbus, OH 43210.

[Haworth co-indexing entry note]: "Considering the Dangers and Opportunities of Pastoral Care and Medicine: A Search for Vitality, Accountability and Balance." Toperzer, Rhoda. Co-published simultaneously in *Journal of Health Care Chaplaincy* (The Haworth Pastoral Press, an imprint of The Haworth Press, Inc.) Vol. 7, No. 1/2, 1998, pp. 117-122; and: *Scientific and Pastoral Perspectives on Intercessory Prayer: An Exchange Between Larry Dossey, M.D. and Health Care Chaplains* (ed: Larry VandeCreek) The Haworth Pastoral Press, an imprint of The Haworth Press, Inc., 1998, pp. 117-122; and: *Scientific and Pastoral Perspectives on Intercessory Prayer: An Exchange Between Larry Dossey, M.D. and Health Care Chaplains* (ed: Larry VandeCreek) Harrington Park Press, an imprint of The Haworth Press, Inc., 1998, pp. 117-122. (Single or multiple copies of this article are available for a fee from The Haworth Document Delivery Service [1-800-342-9678, 9:00 a.m. - 5:00 p.m. (EST). E-mail address: getinfo@haworth.com].

seen if clergy and religious communities will be significant spiritual resources in the years to come or whether they will lose ground.

Perhaps part of the problem lies with the pastoral identity of clergy and religious communities. For many, identity resembles H. Richard Niebuhr's "Christ of Culture" whereby beliefs, behaviors and values stem from what we learn in society. Theological education often exemplifies this through its academic emphasis and benign neglect of spiritual growth in its students.[1] Yet Dossey is part of a shift through spiritualizing medicine toward Neibuhr's "Christ the Transformer of Culture" where the Absolute participates in humanity through "spiritual and natural events" which "are interlocking and analogous."[2] Dossey's expanded definition of prayer as ". . . communication with the Absolute" is compatible with the Judeo-Christian perspective and embraces other religions as well. Chaplains tend to be both personally and professionally receptive to the myriad ways (including appreciation of different world religions) that the "Absolute" is engaged with creation.

Dossey recognizes and appreciates the chaplain's role in the medicine and science relationship. We are comfortable with both science and the sacred; this may be one of our greatest contributions. Those of us in health related pastoral care know the limits and strength of medicine. We are aware that generally "there are no atheists in the hospital" and that people pray for their loved ones especially when there is "nothing else anyone can do." Faith is often evoked/invoked when one is confronted with a medical problem, or when medicine "fails." Chaplains navigate with people through joys and sorrows, strengths and areas of faith which need attention as they make meaning of their experiences.

Spirituality and health research conducted by chaplains is one of the greatest opportunities that follows from Dossey's paper. Trained chaplains with research expertise are in an ideal situation; they possess a theological education, they are comfortable in health care situations and have a clinical population available. Their results contribute to the understanding and practice of wholistic health. Use of the scientific model to confirm and/or refute what we intuitively "know" can lead to new nonmedical or "complementary" practice of care. Pastoral care contributes to research by its unique perspective. When research is critiqued we can attend to criteria which would enhance both design and results as well as hear the existential concerns of our critics. We bring a wholistic paradigm to the research environment; one that can even accept results when we don't know "why?"

Second, pastoral research results can encourage chaplains to overcome false humility and self-inflated tendencies. At the same time, research can promote an accurate picture of our place in the health care field. This can lead to enhanced vitality of our spiritual lives (and facilitate the same among those whom we relate with) as we appreciate the distinctiveness and synergy of body, mind and spirit.

Dossey's commentary about love in the lab suggests an innate human quality that what we study can be approached with love, compassion and curiosity. The opportunity here is to be more vital and imaginative. One does not need to look far to see how the five mainstream religious traditions have their own ways of expressing these qualities. I summarize five major religious traditions.

A Buddhist monk, Thích Nhât Hanh, relects on the Buddhist sacred text, "Heart sutra" and writes about these interconnections within reality.

> The cloud is essential for the paper to exist. If the cloud is not here, the sheet of paper cannot be here either. So we can say the cloud and the paper inter-are. . . . Looking even more deeply, we can see we are in it too. This is not difficult to see, because when we look at a sheet of paper, the sheet of paper is part of our perception. Your mind is in here and mine is also. We can say that everything is in here with this sheet of paper. You cannot point out one thing that is not here–time, space, the rain, the minerals in the soil, the sunshine, the cloud, the river, the heat. Everything coexists with this sheet of paper . . . You cannot just be by yourself alone. You have to inter-be with every other thing. This sheet of paper is, because everything else is.[3]

Christian scripture finds this in Luke where Jesus is challenged to stop people from worship. He responds, "I tell you, if these [people] were silent, the stones would shout."[4]

Sacred Hindu writings reflect on these qualities of love, compassion and curiosity in the Absolute:

> Formless and colorless are you. But in mystery, through your power you transform your light and radiance into many forms and colors in creation. . . . Fill us with the grace of your auspicious thoughts and vision. . . . You are in the woman, in man, you are in the young boy, in the youthful maiden. You are in the old man who walks with his staff. . . . You are in the dark butterfly, in the green parrot with red eyes. . . . You are without beginning, infinite, beyond time and space. All the worlds had their origins in you.[5]

A Judaic scripture draws out "the truth that all things, even the material world, is filled with God's presence. . . . As long as you believe that God is only in heaven and does not fill the earth–let your words be few. . . . when you come to know that you too contain YHWH's presence. . . . then you can pray."[6]

Also, "Under Islam, everything is created by Allah (God) and therefore, everything is sacred, useful and has its place in the general scheme of things and in the interest of man (sic).[7] Clearly this is broad support from the religious arena for honor, respect and celebration of creation. That many scientists see research as a sacred endeavor fits into the *zeitgeist* whereby science and religion aid one another's knowledge. Further, these findings and mystery enhance both disciplines as they both challenge and build upon one another's future.

I now turn to a discussion of three dangers which I experience in Dossey's contribution. *First, though I am grateful that Dossey and other health care providers want to integrate spirituality with their health care practice, their lack of professional training in spirituality may lead to benign, or harmful, medically modeled "spiritual prescriptions."*[8] Chaplains have limits because they do not have a medical education. Physicians have limits because they do not have a theological degree and pastoral care education. Both chaplains and physicians must respect each others' education and professional boundaries. A confounding factor exists; it is that everyone can practice their faith, but all of us are not experts on "disease." Put another way, everyone can practice religion; not everyone is allowed to practice medicine. Conscientious dialogue is needed to avoid these potential pitfalls and to enhance the opportunities of prayer and science.

Second, I am ambivalent about Dossey's challenge to accept parapsychology. This struggle is not one of faith or belief on my part, but pertains to semantics and my knowledge base. I have a bias against that which is labeled "psi phenomena" preferring instead "extra-ordinary awareness" or "intuition." I believe we all have these capacities to some significant extent; we appreciate them or we disregard them. A Gallup study shows that at least one third of the United States population believes in psi phenomena and at least 25% of this population has experienced it.[9] Phenomenologically psi seems to operate much like "faith" experiences which may not be tangibly measured. Both context and community in psi research aid its reputability. As psi continues to be studied with rigorous scientific methodology its validation or refutation furthers our knowledge about science and spirituality.

Third, Dossey's paper lacked any reference to Chinese medicine which has much to contribute to the spirituality/medicine endeavor; I found that startling. It is both rigorously scientific and spiritually based, and not based on emotion.[10] Chinese medicine seeks to assess, diagnose and treat "chi" (energy/life force/spirit). Just as there are various interventions in Western medical care (pills, transfusions, surgery, radiation, etc.), Chinese medicine uses various interventions (herbs, acupuncture, chi balancing, etc.). Asian Indian and Native American medical practice also merit Dossey's consideration. Just as Dossey broadens the definition of prayer, perhaps he can consider the opportunity in Chinese and other integrated forms of medicine to aid the respiritualization of Western medicine.

To conclude, both the vocations of pastoral care and medicine are facing crises in our current cultural settings. Our opportunities are great. Medical and spiritual leadership have shared historical roots; perhaps history needs to teach us professional differentiation before we arrived at this moment, ripe for wholistic cooperation. Perhaps we needed to learn how to look beyond acculturation to learn/diagnose what really ails us in order to access what can heal us. This is a time for rich dialogue amongst ourselves and with the medical profession if we are to, prophetically and with collegiality, claim our strengths and learn from one another. Borrowing from the philosophy of Chinese medicine, chi seeks balance among very different and related qualities, or elements which vary in their receptivity to one another according to the moment. Perhaps pastoral care and medicine can help one another as we seek balance of body and spirit, of science and prayer, thereby enriching both.

REFERENCES

1. Samuel Calian Carnegie. "Prayer during seminary years and beyond." *Perspectives* 1995; 16-18.

2. H. Richard Niebuhr. *Christ and Culture* (New York: Harper and Row, 1951), 197.

3. Thích Nhât Hanh. *The Heart of Understanding* (Berkeley, California: Parallax Press, 1988), 3-4.

4. Luke 19:39-40, 83.

5. Joel Beverluis, editor. *A Sourcebook for the Community of Religions* (Chicago: The Council for a Parliament of World's Religions, 1993), 65.

6. Arthur Green and Barry W. Holtz. *Your Word Is Fire: The Hasidic Masters on Contemplative Prayer* (New York: Schocken Books, 1977), 31.

7. Joel Beverluis, 154.

8. Keith Wall. "Prescription: Prayer." *Physician* January/February 1994; 17.

9. George Gallup. Lecture at Harvard Medical School Conference on Spirituality and Healing, December 3, 1995.

10. David Eisenberger, MD, with Thomas Lee Wright. *Encounters With Qi: Exploring Chinese Medicine* (New York: Penguin Books, 1985).

CURRENT CONTENTS
IN THE LITERATURE OF INTEREST
TO PASTORAL CARE

Introduction

W. Noel Brown, Editor

Prayer is an important activity in the daily life of a majority of Americans. It is an activity that people expect chaplains to engage in. And so it is not surprising that in the pastoral care literature there is a steady stream of articles on the subject. What is surprising is the recent upsurge in interest in prayer and meditation and how these activities can affect health and well-being. Further, they are now subjects which can be the occasion of serious research, reported in peer-reviewed journals. But that is not all, a small, but growing number of doctors and nurses are discussing how they should pray with their patients.

W. Noel Brown is affiliated with the Department of Religion and Health (MC-2120), University of Chicago Hospitals, 5841 South Maryland Avenue, Chicago, IL 60617 (E-mail: Noel_Brown_at_OPR-2@mcis.bsd.uchicago.edu).

[Haworth co-indexing entry note]: "Introduction." Brown, W. Noel. Co-published simultaneously in *Journal of Health Care Chaplaincy* (The Haworth Pastoral Press, an imprint of The Haworth Press, Inc.) Vol. 7, No. 1/2, 1998, pp. 123-135; and: *Scientific and Pastoral Perspectives on Intercessory Prayer: An Exchange Between Larry Dossey, M.D. and Health Care Chaplains* (ed: Larry VandeCreek) The Haworth Pastoral Press, an imprint of The Haworth Press, Inc., 1998, pp. 123-135; and: *Scientific and Pastoral Perspectives on Intercessory Prayer: An Exchange Between Larry Dossey, M.D. and Health Care Chaplains* (ed: Larry VandeCreek) Harrington Park Press, an imprint of The Haworth Press, Inc., 1998, pp. 123-135. Single or multiple copies of this article are available for a fee from The Haworth Document Delivery Service [1-800-342-9678, 9:00 a.m. - 5:00 p.m. (EST). E-mail address: getinfo@haworth.com].

123

In making this review of the journal literature concerning prayer and meditation, a search was conducted going back to 1990. While the pastoral care literature was the primary focus, an additional search of the medical, nursing and psychological journals was also conducted. It produced some interesting results.

Some earlier papers have been included because of their historical importance. From some of the titles, it may not be immediately apparent that the subject of meditation or prayer is mentioned in the article itself. The search involved examining the articles themselves to ensure that prayer and meditation were included topics.

The articles have been grouped into four sections though with difficulty in some cases because an article straddles the line between several topics, and could have been included in another section.

The Use of Prayer in Pastoral Care and Counseling

William A. Barry
Prayer in pastoral care: a contribution from the tradition
of spiritual direction
Journal of Pastoral Care
Volume 31 # 2 (June 1977)
Pages 91-96

Katy Butler
"Pray without ceasing"
Common Boundary
Volume 9 # 6 (Nov/Dec 1991)
Pages 33-35

Donald Capps
Praying in our own behalf: toward the revitalization
of petitionary prayer
Second Opinion
Volume 19 # 1 (July 1993)
Pages 21-40

Bruce Evanson, Elaine Goodell, Geaorge F. Handzo
and Stephen Shulman
Prayer and pastoral care
The CareGiver Journal

Volume 10 # 3 (1993)
Pages 40-47

Karl F. Fickling
Leading group meditations for recovering patients
Journal of Health Care Chaplaincy
Volume 3 # 1 (1990)
Pages 41-52

George L. Hogben, Kathleen Keefe, and Richard O'Gorman
Prayer and Catholic sacramental practice in the treatment of a case
of psychosis
Journal of Christian Healing
Volume 16 # 2 (Summer 1994)
Pages 16-21

Monica A. Lucas
Praying with the terminally ill
Journal of Health Care Chaplaincy
Volume 6 # 1 (1994)
Pages 61-71

Paul A. Mandziuk
Easing chronic pain with spiritual resources
Journal of Religion and Health
Volume 32 # 1 (Spring 1993)
Pages 47-54

Jessica Rose
A needle-quivering poise: Between prayer and practice
in the counseling relationship
Contact Monograph
Volume 6 (1996)
Pages 2-36

Karyn L. Shadbolt
Ministering to families in chronic crisis: soulwork: healing
Ministry
Volume 4 # 3 (May/June 1997)
Pages 24-28

Henry C. Simmons
"Teach us to pray": pastoral care of the new nursing home resident
Journal of Pastoral Care
Volume 45 # 2 (Summer 1991)
Pages 169-176

Wendy M. Wright
Seasons of glad songs: entries from a notebook on scripture
and prayer
Weavings
Volume 11 # 4 (July/Aug 1996)
Pages 6-15

Research into the Use of Prayer/Meditation and Their Effects

Lucille B. Bearon, and Harold G. Koenig
Religious cognitions and use of prayer in health and illness
The Gerontologist
Volume 30 # 2 (1990)
Pages 249-253

Marion A. Bilich and Steven D. Carlson
Therapist and clergy working together: linking the psychological
with the spiritual in the treatment of MPD
Journal of Christian Healing
Volume 16 # 1 (Spring 1994)
Pages 3-11

Randolph C. Byrd
Positive therapeutic effects of intercessory prayer in a coronary care unit
Southern Medical Journal
Volume 81 # 7 (July 1988)
Pages 826-829

Platon J. Collipp
The efficacy of prayer: a triple blind study
Medical Times
Volume 97 # 5 (May 1969)
Pages 201-4

Jagdish K. Dua and Michelle L. Swinden
Effectiveness of negative-thought-reduction, meditation, and placebo
Scandinavian Journal of Psychology
Volume 33 # 1 (Jan 1992)
Pages 135-146

Paul N. Duckro and Philip R. Magaletta
The effect of prayer on physical health: experimental evidence
Journal of Religion and Health
Volume 33 # 3 (Fall 1994)
Pages 211-220

Julia Emblen and Lois Halstead
Spiritual needs and interventions: comparing the views
of patients, nurses
Clinical Nurse Specialist
Volume 7 # 4 (1993)
Pages 175-182

L. J. Francis
Personality and prayer among adult churchgoers: a replication
Social Behavior and Personality
Volume 24 # 4 (1996)
Pages 405-407

Paul Fulton
Psychologists study prayer and other religious topics
Common Boundary
Volume 9 # 3 (July/Aug 1991)
Pages 39-40

C. R. B. Joyce and R. M. C. Welldon
The objective efficacy of prayer: a double-blind clinical trial
Journal of Chronic Disease
Volume 18 # 1 (April 1965)
Pages 367-377

Jon Kabat-Zinn, Ann O. Massion, Jean Kristeller,
Linda G. Peterson et al.
Effectiveness of a meditation-based stress reduction program

in the treatment of anxiety disorders
American Journal of Psychiatry
Volume 149 # 7 (July 1992)
Pages 936-943

P. M. Lehrer
Varieties of relaxation methods and their unique effects
International Journal of Stress Management
Volume 3 # 1 (Jan 1996)
Pages 1-15

J. K. Lepuschitz
Meditation and psychosocial adaptation: an exploratory study
Current Psychology
Volume 15 # 3 (Fall 1996)
Pages 283-329

Jeffrey S. Levin, J. S. Lyons, and D. B. Larson
Prayer and health during pregnancy: findings from the Galveston low birth weight study
Southern Medical Journal
Volume 86 # 9 (1993)
Pages 1022-1027

Jeffrey S. Levin and P. L. Schiller
Is there a religious factor in health?
Journal of Religion and Health
Volume 267 (1987)
Pages 9-36

JoAnn O'Reilly
A community of strangers: finding solidarity through prayer request
Care Give Journal
Volume 11 # 2 (1994-1995)
Pages 26-30

Margaret M. Poloma
The effects of prayer of mental well-being
Second Opinion
Volume 18 # 3 (Jan 1993)
Pages 37-51

Margaret M. Poloma
Evidence of prayer's healing power: a sociological perspective
Second Opinion
Volume 20 # 1 (July 1994)
Pages 82-85

Wade Roush
Herbert Benson: mind-body maverick pushes the envelope
Science
Volume 276 # 5311 (18 Apr 1997)
Pages 357-359

Theresa L. Saudia, Marguerite R. Kinney, Kathleen C. Brown
and Leslie Young-Ward
Health locus of control and helpfulness of prayer
Heart and Lung
Volume 20 # 1 (Jan 1991)
Pages 60-65

Marilyn S. Saur and William G. Saur
Transitional phenomena as evidenced in prayer
Journal of Religion and Health
Volume 32 # 1 (Spring 1993)
Pages 55-66

Susanne Schneider and Robert Kastenbaum
Patterns and meanings of prayer in hospice caregivers:
an exploratory study
Death Studies
Volume 17 # 6 (Nov/Dec 1993)
Pages 471-486

A. C. Tjeltveit
Relationships among mental health values and various dimensions
of religiousness
Journal of Social and Clinical Psychology
Volume 15 # 3 (Fall 1996)
Pages 364-377

Keith S. Thomson
The revival of experiments on prayer
American Scientist
Volume 84 # 6 (Nov/Dec 1996)
Pages 532-534

Ferris B. Urbanowski and John J. Miller
Trauma, psychotherapy and meditation
Journal of Transpersonal Psychology
Volume 28 # 1 (Jan 1996)
Pages 31-48

Charles Zeiders and Ronald J. Pekala
A review of the evidence regarding the behavioral, medical
and psychological efficacy of Christian prayer
Journal of Christian Healing
Volume 17 # 3 (Fall 1995)
Pages 17-27

Understanding the Place of Prayer/Meditation in Health

Richard Bellingham, Barry Cohen, Todd Jones and LeRoy Spaniol
Connectedness: some skills for spiritual health
American J. of Health Promotion
Volume 4 # 1 (Sept/Oct 1989)
Pages 18-24, 31

Susan Blackmore
Is meditation good for you?
New Scientist
Volume 131 # 1776 (July 6 1991)
Pages 30-33

Larry Dossey
Healing words
Psychological Perspectives
Volume 28 (Fall/Winter 1993)
Pages 20-31

Larry Dossey
Can prayer harm?
Psychology Today
Volume 30 # 2 (Mar/Apr 1997)
Pages 49-52, 75, 76

Christopher G. Ellison and Robert J. Taylor
Turning to prayer: social and situational antecedents
of religious coping
Review of Religious Research
Volume 38 # 2 (Dec 1996)
Pages 111-117

Bruce G. Epperly
To pray or not to pray: reflections on the intersection of prayer
and medicine
Journal of Religion and Health
Volume 34 # 2 (Summer 1995)
Pages 141-148

Nancy Flam
Healing the Spirit: a Jewish approach
Cross Currents
(Winter 1996/7)
Pages 487-497

Daniel Goleman and Joel Gurin
Mind/body medicine–at last
Psychology Today
Volume 26 # 2 (Mar/Apr 1993)
Pages 16, 80

Virginia S. Harris
Christian Science spiritual healing practices
The Christian Science Journal
Volume 115 # 3 (Mar 1997)
Pages 20-26

Jon Kabat-Zinn
Meditate !–for stress reduction, inner peace. . . .
Psychology Today
Volume 26 # 4 (July/Aug 1993)
Pages 37-41, 68-69

Harold G. Koenig, Lucille B. Bearon and Richard Dayringer
Physician perspectives on the role of religion
in the patient relationship
Journal of Family Practise
Volume 28 # 4 (Apr 1989)
Pages 441-448

Harold G. Koenig, J. C. Hays, L. K. George, D. G. Blazer,
David B. Larson, and L. R. Landerman
Modeling the cross-sectional relationships between religion,
physical health, social support and depressive symptoms
American Journal of Geriatric Psychiatry
Volume 5 # 2 (1997)
Pages 131-144

Jeffrey S. Levin
How religion influences morbidity and health: reflections on natural
history, salutogenesis and host resistance
Social Science and Medicine
Volume 43 # 5 (1996)
Pages 849-864

Michael E. McCullough
Prayer and health: conceptual issues, research review,
and research agenda
Journal of Psychology and Theology
Volume 23 # 1 (Spring 1995)
Pages 15-30

Ernest L. Rossi
Do we really have a prayer?
Psychological Perspectives
Volume 28 (Fall/Winter 1993)
Pages 6-19

David Ruben
Meditation goes mainstream
New Age Journal
Volume 8 # 3 (May/June 1991)
Pages 42-45, 112

Walter J. Smith
The role of mental health in spiritual growth
Journal of Religion in Disability and Rehabilitation
Volume 1 # 2 (1994)
Pages 27-40

The Use of Prayer by Physicians and Nurses

Teo Forcht Dagi
Prayer, picty, and professional propriety: limits
on religious expression
Journal of Clinical Ethics
Volume 6 # 3 (Fall 1995)
Pages 274-279

Rodur Gabuya
Interview with Dr. Jarad Kass
Journal of Health Care Chaplaincy
Volume 3 # 1 (1990)
Pages 81-91

H. Phil Gross
Is it appropriate to pray in the operating room?
Journal of Clinical Ethics
Volume 6 # 3 (Fall 1995)
Pages 273-274

Pamela J. Lewis
A review of prayer within the role of the holistic nurse
Journal of Holistic Nursing
Volume 14 # 4 (Dec 1996)
Pages 308-315

Philip R. Magaletta and Paul N. Duckro
Prayer in the medical encounter
Journal of Religion and Health
Volume 35 # 3 (Fall 1996)
Pages 203-209

Philip R. Magaletta, Paul N. Duckro and Stephen F. Staten
Prayer in office practice: on the threshold of integration
Journal of Family Practice
Volume 44 # 3 (Mar 1997)
Pages 254-256

Charles Marwick
Should physicians prescribe prayer for health? Spiritual aspects
of well-being considered
JAMA
Volume 273 # 20 (24/31 May 1995)
Pages 1561-1562

Gary Thomas
Doctors who pray
Christianity Today
Volume 41 # 1 (6 Jan 1997)
Pages 20-30

General

Graeme Chapman
When Christians pray
Ministry Society and Theology
Volume 10 # 2 (Nov 1996)
Pages 10-18

Janet M. Kamer
My personal experience with deliverance prayer
Journal of Christian Healing
Volume 17 # 4 (Winter 1995)
Pages 26-28

Tom Kavanagh
Between heaven and earth
Common Boundary
Volume 13 # 1 (Jan/Feb 1995)
Pages 44-49

Patrick D. Miller
Prayer as persuasion: the rhetoric and intention of prayer
Word and World
Volume 13 # 4 (Fall 1993)
Pages 356-362

Anne A. Simpkinson
Resting in God
Common Boundary
Volume 15 # 3 (Sept/Oct 1997)
Pages 24 31

James Woodward
Divine action, Christian belief and prayer
Contact
Volume 112 (1993)
Pages 13-21

Subject Index

Index of Names and Titles

(Does not include materials in the "Current Contents in the Literature of Interest to Pastoral Care" found at the end of this volume)

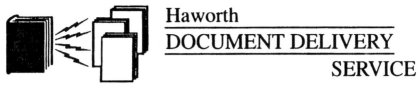

Haworth
DOCUMENT DELIVERY
SERVICE

This valuable service provides a single-article order form for any article from a Haworth journal.

- *Time Saving:* No running around from library to library to find a specific article.
- *Cost Effective:* All costs are kept down to a minimum.
- *Fast Delivery:* Choose from several options, including same-day FAX.
- *No Copyright Hassles:* You will be supplied by the original publisher.
- *Easy Payment:* Choose from several easy payment methods.

Open Accounts Welcome for . . .
- Library Interlibrary Loan Departments
- Library Network/Consortia Wishing to Provide Single-Article Services
- Indexing/Abstracting Services with Single Article Provision Services
- Document Provision Brokers and Freelance Information Service Providers

---

MAIL or FAX THIS ENTIRE ORDER FORM TO:

Haworth Document Delivery Service
The Haworth Press, Inc.
10 Alice Street
Binghamton, NY 13904-1580

or FAX: 1-800-895-0582
or CALL: 1-800-342-9678
9am-5pm EST

PLEASE SEND ME PHOTOCOPIES OF THE FOLLOWING SINGLE ARTICLES:
1) Journal Title: _____
   Vol/Issue/Year: _____ Starting & Ending Pages: _____
   Article Title: _____
   _____

2) Journal Title: _____
   Vol/Issue/Year: _____ Starting & Ending Pages: _____
   Article Title: _____
   _____

3) Journal Title: _____
   Vol/Issue/Year: _____ Starting & Ending Pages: _____
   Article Title: _____
   _____

4) Journal Title: _____
   Vol/Issue/Year: _____ Starting & Ending Pages: _____
   Article Title: _____
   _____

(See other side for Costs and Payment Information)

COSTS: Please figure your cost to order quality copies of an article.

1. Set-up charge per article: $8.00
   ($8.00 × number of separate articles)   _____

2. Photocopying charge for each article:

   1-10 pages: $1.00   _____

   11-19 pages: $3.00   _____

   20-29 pages: $5.00   _____

   30+ pages: $2.00/10 pages   _____

3. Flexicover (optional): $2.00/article   _____

4. Postage & Handling: US: $1.00 for the first article/
   $.50 each additional article   _____

   Federal Express: $25.00   _____

   Outside US: $2.00 for first article/
   $.50 each additional article_____

5. Same-day FAX service: $.35 per page   _____

GRAND TOTAL: _____

METHOD OF PAYMENT: (please check one)

❑ Check enclosed   ❑ Please ship and bill. PO # _____
(sorry we can ship and bill to bookstores only! All others must pre-pay)

❑ Charge to my credit card: ❑ Visa; ❑ MasterCard; ❑ Discover;
❑ American Express;

Account Number:_____ Expiration date:_____

Signature: ✗_____

Name: _____ Institution: _____

Address: _____

_____

City: _____ State:_____ Zip:_____

Phone Number: _____ FAX Number: _____

MAIL or *FAX* THIS ENTIRE ORDER FORM TO:

Haworth Document Delivery Service	**or FAX:** 1-800-895-0582
The Haworth Press, Inc.	**or CALL:** 1-800-342-9678
10 Alice Street	9am-5pm EST)
Binghamton, NY 13904-1580	